OTH[

Fast Facts A[ ]nals (*Adams*)

Fast Facts fo[ ]now in a Nutshell, Sec[

Fast Facts for the ER NURSE: Emergency Department Orientation in a Nutshell, Third Edition (*Buettner*)

Fast Facts About GI AND LIVER DISEASES FOR NURSES: What APRNs Need to Know in a Nutshell (*Chaney*)

Fast Facts for the MEDICAL–SURGICAL NURSE: Clinical Orientation in a Nutshell (*Ciocco*)

Fast Facts on COMBATING NURSE BULLYING, INCIVILITY, AND WORKPLACE VIOLENCE: What Nurses Need to Know in a Nutshell (*Ciocco*)

Fast Facts for the NURSE PRECEPTOR: Keys to Providing a Successful Preceptorship in a Nutshell (*Ciocco*)

Fast Facts for the OPERATING ROOM NURSE: An Orientation and Care Guide, Second Edition (*Criscitelli*)

Fast Facts for the ANTEPARTUM AND POSTPARTUM NURSE: A Nursing Orientation and Care Guide in a Nutshell (*Davidson*)

Fast Facts for the NEONATAL NURSE: A Nursing Orientation and Care Guide in a Nutshell (*Davidson*)

Fast Facts Workbook for CARDIAC DYSRHYTHMIAS AND 12-LEAD EKGs (*Desmarais*)

Fast Facts About PRESSURE ULCER CARE FOR NURSES: How to Prevent, Detect, and Resolve Them in a Nutshell (*Dziedzic*)

Fast Facts for the GERONTOLOGY NURSE: A Nursing Care Guide in a Nutshell (*Eliopoulos*)

Fast Facts for the LONG-TERM CARE NURSE: What Nursing Home and Assisted Living Nurses Need to Know in a Nutshell (*Eliopoulos*)

Fast Facts for the CLINICAL NURSE MANAGER: Managing a Changing Workplace in a Nutshell, Second Edition (*Fry*)

Fast Facts for EVIDENCE-BASED PRACTICE IN NURSING: Implementing EBP in a Nutshell, Second Edition (*Godshall*)

Fast Facts for Nurses About HOME INFUSION THERAPY: The Expert's Best Practice Guide in a Nutshell (*Gorski*)

Fast Facts About NURSING AND THE LAW: Law for Nurses in a Nutshell (*Grant, Ballard*)

Fast Facts for the L&D NURSE: Labor & Delivery Orientation in a Nutshell, Second Edition (*Groll*)

Fast Facts for the RADIOLOGY NURSE: An Orientation and Nursing Care Guide in a Nutshell (*Grossman*)

Fast Facts on ADOLESCENT HEALTH FOR NURSING AND HEALTH PROFESSIONALS: A Care Guide in a Nutshell (*Herrman*)

Fast Facts for the FAITH COMMUNITY NURSE: Implementing FCN/Parish Nursing in a Nutshell (*Hickman*)

Fast Facts for the CARDIAC SURGERY NURSE: Caring for Cardiac Surgery Patients in a Nutshell, Second Edition (*Hodge*)

Fast Facts About the NURSING PROFESSION: Historical Perspectives in a Nutshell (*Hunt*)

Fast Facts for the CLINICAL NURSING INSTRUCTOR: Clinical Teaching in a Nutshell, Third Edition (*Kan, Stabler-Haas*)

Fast Facts for the WOUND CARE NURSE: Practical Wound Management in a Nutshell (*Kifer*)

Fast Facts About EKGs FOR NURSES: The Rules of Identifying EKGs in a Nutshell (*Landrum*)

Fast Facts for the CRITICAL CARE NURSE: Critical Care Nursing in a Nutshell (*Landrum*)

Fast Facts for the TRAVEL NURSE: Travel Nursing in a Nutshell (*Landrum*)

Fast Facts for the SCHOOL NURSE: School Nursing in a Nutshell, Second Edition (*Loschiavo*)

Fast Facts for MANAGING PATIENTS WITH A PSYCHIATRIC DISORDER: What RNs, NPs, and New Psych Nurses Need to Know (*Marshall*)

Fast Facts About SUBSTANCE USE DISORDERS: What Every Nurse, APRN, and PA Needs to Know (*Marshall, Spencer*)

Fast Facts About CURRICULUM DEVELOPMENT IN NURSING: How to Develop and Evaluate Educational Programs in a Nutshell, Second Edition (*McCoy, Anema*)

Fast Facts for the CATH LAB NURSE (*McCulloch*)

Fast Facts About NEUROCRITICAL CARE: A Quick Reference for the Advanced Practice Provider (*McLaughlin*)

Fast Facts for DEMENTIA CARE: What Nurses Need to Know in a Nutshell (*Miller*)

Fast Facts for HEALTH PROMOTION IN NURSING: Promoting Wellness in a Nutshell (*Miller*)

Fast Facts for STROKE CARE NURSING: An Expert Care Guide, Second Edition (*Morrison*)

Fast Facts for the MEDICAL OFFICE NURSE: What You Really Need to Know in a Nutshell (*Richmeier*)

Fast Facts for the PEDIATRIC NURSE: An Orientation Guide in a Nutshell (*Rupert, Young*)

Fast Facts About FORENSIC NURSING: What You Need to Know (*Scannell*)

Fast Facts About the GYNECOLOGICAL EXAM: A Professional Guide for NPs, PAs, and Midwives, Second Edition (*Secor, Fantasia*)

Fast Facts for the STUDENT NURSE: Nursing Student Success in a Nutshell (*Stabler-Haas*)

Fast Facts for CAREER SUCCESS IN NURSING: Making the Most of Mentoring in a Nutshell (*Vance*)

Fast Facts for the TRIAGE NURSE: An Orientation and Care Guide, Second Edition (*Visser, Montejano*)

Fast Facts for DEVELOPING A NURSING ACADEMIC PORTFOLIO: What You Really Need to Know in a Nutshell (*Wittmann-Price*)

Fast Facts for the HOSPICE NURSE: A Concise Guide to End-of-Life Care (*Wright*)

Fast Facts for the CLASSROOM NURSING INSTRUCTOR: Classroom Teaching in a Nutshell (*Yoder-Wise, Kowalski*)

Forthcoming FAST FACTS Books

Fast Facts About NEUROPATHIC PAIN (*Davies*)

Fact Facts in HEALTH INFORMATICS FOR NURSES (*Hardy*)

Fact Facts About NURSE ANESTHESIA (*Hickman*)

Fast Facts for the CARDIAC SURGERY NURSE, Third Edition (*Hodge*)

Fast Facts for the CRITICAL CARE NURSE: Critical Care Nursing, Second Edition (*Landrum*)

Fast Facts for the SCHOOL NURSE, Third Edition (*Loschiavo*)

Fast Facts on How to Conduct, Understand, and Maybe Even Love RESEARCH! For Nurses and Other Healthcare Providers (*Marshall*)

Fast Facts About RELIGION FOR NURSES: Implications for Patient Care (*Taylor*)

Visit www.springerpub.com to order.

FAST FACTS About
FORENSIC NURSING

Meredith J. Scannell, PhD, MSN, MPH, CNM, SANE-A, CEN, is currently an assistant professor at the Massachusetts General Hospital (MGH) Institute of Health Professions and a staff nurse in the Center for Clinical Investigation and the Emergency Department at the Brigham and Women's Hospital in Boston, Massachusetts. She received her certification as a sexual assault nurse examiner (SANE) in 2004 and is currently employed as a SANE in the Massachusetts Department of Public Health, conducting forensic examinations and evidence collection at seven Boston area hospitals. Dr. Scannell has published numerous articles on violence against women and women's health and continues her research focus in HIV postexposure prophylaxis in the sexually assaulted individuals. She has developed a simulation course titled Sexual Assault Simulation Course for Healthcare Providers (SASH), which is an interprofessional course for nurses, doctors, and physician assistants in how to deliver care to sexually assaulted patients. She is also certified as a nurse midwife and has published on various topics related to pregnant women, and she has presented national and internationally on various topics.

FAST FACTS About
FORENSIC NURSING

What You Need to Know

Meredith J. Scannell, PhD, MSN, MPH, CNM, SANE-A, CEN

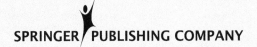
SPRINGER PUBLISHING COMPANY

Springer Publishing Company, LLC
11 West 42nd Street
New York, NY 10036
www.springerpub.com

Acquisitions Editor: Margaret Zuccarini
Compositor: Amnet Systems

ISBN: 978-0-8261-3866-8
e-book ISBN: 978-0-8261-3867-5

18 19 20 21 22 / 5 4 3 2 1

The author and the publisher of this Work have made every effort to use sources believed to be reliable to provide information that is accurate and compatible with the standards generally accepted at the time of publication. The author and publisher shall not be liable for any special, consequential, or exemplary damages resulting, in whole or in part, from the readers' use of, or reliance on, the information contained in this book. The publisher has no responsibility for the persistence or accuracy of URLs for external or third-party Internet websites referred to in this publication and does not guarantee that any content on such websites is, or will remain, accurate or appropriate.

Library of Congress Cataloging-in-Publication Data
Names: Scannell, Meredith J., author.
Title: Fast facts about forensic nursing : what you need to know / [edited
  by] Meredith J. Scannell.
Other titles: Fast facts (Springer Publishing Company)
Description: New York, NY : Springer Publishing Company, LLC, [2019] |
  Series: Fast facts | Includes bibliographical references and index.
Identifiers: LCCN 2018042113| ISBN 9780826138668 (print : alk. paper) | ISBN
  9780826138675 (ebook)
Subjects: | MESH: Forensic Nursing
Classification: LCC RA1053 | NLM WY 170 | DDC 614/.1—dc23
LC record available at https://lccn.loc.gov/2018042113

Contact us to receive discount rates on bulk purchases.
We can also customize our books to meet your needs.
For more information, please contact sales@springerpub.com

Publisher's Note: New and used products purchased from third-party sellers are not guaranteed for quality, authenticity, or access to any included digital components.

Printed in the United States of America.

Contents

Contributors

Stacy Brady, MSN, APRN, CCRN, ACCNS-AG

Critical Care Clinical Nurse Specialist; Emergency Department Staff Nurse
Providence Veterans Affairs Medical Center; Brigham and Women's Hospital
Providence, Rhode Island; Boston, Massachusetts

George E. Flores, MS, RN

Commander, U.S. Public Health Service
Senior Staff Nurse, Emergency Department
Alaska Native Medical Center
Anchorage, Alaska

Corrine Foster, BS, ADN, RN, CFRN, CCRN, CEN, C-NPT, EMT

Trauma Critical Care Team Nurse, National Disaster Medical System
Critical Care Flight Nurse, Boston Medflight
Emergency Department Staff Nurse, Forensic Liaison, Brigham and Women's Hospital
Boston, Massachusetts

Yaeko Marie Karantonis, BSN, RN

Staff Nurse; Clinical Supervisory Nurse
Brigham and Women's Hospital; National Disaster Medical System
Boston, Massachusetts

Andrea MacDonald, MSN/MBA, RN, SANE-A

Staff Nurse, Forensic Liaison
Brigham and Women's Hospital Emergency Department
Boston, Massachusetts

Barbara P. Madden, EdD, RN

Professor Emerita, Fitchburg State University
Sexual Assault Nurse Examiner, Massachusetts Department of Public Health
Boston, Massachusetts

Diane L. Miller, MSN, RN, ACNS, CEN

Professional Development
  Manager
Brigham and Women's Hospital
Boston, Massachusetts

Patricia A. Normandin, DNP, RN, CEN, CPN, CPEN, FAEN

Staff Nurse and Nurse Scientist,
  Tufts Medical Center Emergency
  Department
Adjunct Nursing Faculty,
  Massachusetts General Hospital
  Institute of Health Professions
Boston, Massachusetts

Kristine Ruggiero, PhD, MSN, RN, CPNP

Pediatric Nurse Practitioner and
  Nurse Scientist, Boston Children's
  Hospital
Assistant Professor of Nursing,
  Massachusetts General Hospital
  Institute of Health Professions
Boston, Massachusetts

Preface

Forensic nursing is a growing nursing field blending nursing science with forensic science, law, and criminology. A forensic nurse is one who provides specialized care for patients who are victims and perpetrators in medicolegal cases. At its core, this specialty seeks to address healthcare issues that have a medicolegal component that often involves violence, trauma, death, abuses, criminal activity, liability, and accidents. Forensic nurses trained in this field have enhanced education and training in the forensic practices of documenting injuries, collecting biological fluids, and preserving evidence such as clothing from the assault. Forensic nurses often act as multidisciplinary team members from various healthcare settings and law enforcement as well. Knowing foundational aspects of forensic nursing can serve nurses who care for diverse patients and may be victims of abuse or crimes. Forensic nurses have a unique lens that enables them to detect whether their patients are being subjected to inhumane treatment or not and give the best treatment to them and provide linkage to services. Forensic nursing is vital to patient care and, to some degree, nurses in almost any clinical setting will use forensic nursing skills in screening, assessing, and treating patients. This book provides insight into some common and not-so-common aspects of forensic nursing and how nurses in any setting can implement forensic nursing skills in delivering optimal care to patients.

Meredith J. Scannell,
PhD, MSN, MPH, CNM, SANE-A, CEN

I

Overview of Forensic Nursing Principles and Practice

1

History of Forensic Nursing

Meredith J. Scannell

Forensic nursing is a subspecialty of nursing that involves the application of forensic science and nursing. It has been incorporated in various healthcare areas, including hospitals, emergency departments (EDs), healthcare clinics, legal practices, correctional institutions, psychiatric institutions, public health organizations, correctional facilities, coroners' offices, school systems, and other organizations and healthcare environments. Forensic nurses may also be involved with mass disasters and community crisis situations, applying a forensic lens to various clinical and practice settings.

At the end of the chapter, the nurse will be able to:

1. Understand the history of forensic nursing and the role of the forensic nurse.
2. List the different educational methods in achieving different forensic nursing degrees.
3. Recognize past forensic nursing pioneers and their contribution to the forensic nursing community.

BACKGROUND

The inception of forensics and medicine has been noted to go back as far as the days of early civilization, with evidence suggesting Egyptian and Hindu medicine showed an understanding of poisons and toxicology (Smith, 1951). Greek civilization and Hippocrates would discuss injury patterns as well as an understanding and an oath of not using poisons. The Romans used injury pattern identification in determining the cause of death, such as in the case of Julius Caesar (Smith, 1951). Ancient Chinese documents also revealed evidence in medical death investigations and wound identifications (Smith, 1951). It was only natural for forensics to find its way into nursing.

Published documents have demonstrated clear forensic nursing practice in the United Kingdom in the 1950s (Smith, 1951). In the United Kingdom, healthcare professionals, including nurses, often formed partnerships with law enforcement so that they could provide healthcare and forensic medicine to those in the custody of law enforcement and within the "custodial environment" (Officer, 1979). The role was specific to individuals with mental health and substance use disorders or dealt with child sexual assault (Officer, 1979). Other clinical duties included obtaining medical histories, administering medications, assessing mental health, determining the individual's ability to be interviewed, providing reports to law enforcement, giving court testimony, and appearing as a fact or expert witness (Officer, 1979). Some of the responsibilities would be included after the nurse had additional training and experience in making precise injury documentation and forensic interpretation, taking forensic samples and giving an opinion on suspicious deaths, and conducting examinations of victims (adults and children) of sexual assault. In other healthcare systems, forensic nursing derived from mental health where it was known as "forensic psychiatry" and patients were often referred to as "forensic patients" who were on "forensic units" and were involved in the criminal justice system (Galappathie, Khan, & Hussain, 2017).

Earliest documented aspects of forensic nursing in the United States date back to the 1970s (Speck & Aiken, 1995; Clark, 1976). Much of the forensic nursing involved nursing and victims of sexual assault (Clark, 1976). Nurse Ann Burgess and sociologist Lynda Holstrom conducted extensive research with victims of sexual assault and developed the rape trauma syndrome and treatment for victims of sexual assault (Burgess & Holstrom, 1985). Nurses worked in sexual assault centers that were established during this period. They were also often the ones who counseled victims of assault, helped to navigate their emergency visit, and offered advice and support during the initial encounter and follow-up care. Formal recognition of forensic nursing began in the early 1980s, largely from the work done by Virginal Lynch (Lynch & Duval, 2011). The Scope and Standards of Forensic Nursing Practice was first developed to help standardize the practice of forensic nursing, shortly after the International Association of Forensic Nurses (IAFN) was created. Forensic nursing in the United States was established in death investigations and soon made its way into different aspects of nursing where there are specialized forensic nurses with different degrees and certification.

NOTABLE FORENSIC NURSES

Ann Wolbert Burgess

Ann Wolbert Burgess, DNSc, APRN, FAAN, is one of the most notable forensic nurse researchers. She is internationally known for her work on topics related to sexual assault and interpersonal violence. One of her most notable works of research in 1974 with sociologist Lynda Lytle Holstrom was on rape victimology, and it led to the development of the rape trauma syndrome (Burgess & Holmstrom, 1985). "Rape trauma syndrome" is a term that refers to a myriad of reactions and responses a victim of sexual assault will have (Burgess & Holmstrom, 1985). This work gave insight into the perspective of the victims and has been the foundation of various other works of research. Dr. Burgess also worked closely with the Behavioral Science Unit of the Federal Bureau of Investigation (FBI) in developing the psychological profiling of perpetrators. She has authored numerous books and journal articles and was named by the American Academy of Nursing as a living legend, and she has received various honors, including the Sigma Theta Tau International Audrey Hepburn Award, the American Nurses Association Hildegard Peplau Award, and the Sigma Theta Tau International Episteme Laureate Award.

Virginia Lynch

Virginia Lynch is considered one of the founders and authorities on forensic nursing and forensic science (Maguire & Raso, 2017). She was fundamental in the creation of the forensic nursing specialty and instrumental in developing the standards for forensic nursing, which have paved the way in promoting health and justice worldwide (Maguire & Raso, 2017). In the 1980s she developed the forensic nursing curriculum and forensic nursing model. She was the first president of the IAFN and has received numerous awards for her work, and she is considered one of the founding members of forensic nursing, which is illustrated in the highest and prestigious award given by the IAFN, titled the Virginia A. Lynch Pioneer Award in Forensic Nursing. She has authored numerous books, detailing the science of forensic nursing (Lynch & Duval, 2011).

Education for forensic nurses includes some of the following topics:

- Trauma-informed care
- Forensic interview
- Forensic photography
- Identification of different types of abuse, including physical, psychological, sexual, and economic
- Assessment and documentation of wounds
- Identification of defensive wounds
- Interpretation of blunt, sharp, penetrating trauma
- Evidence collection
- Jurisprudence
- Topics specific to interpersonal violence, including child maltreatment, elder abuse, sexual abuse, and human trafficking
- Death investigations
- Biological evidence and DNA testing and analysis
- Mass disasters and community crises

FORENSIC NURSING

In several clinical settings, nurses use forensic skills with are often not identified as forensic yet have their roots in forensic science. Forensic nursing is practiced by nurses who work in different clinical settings, such as hospital, schools, correctional institutions, and mental and psychiatric healthcare settings (Lynch & Duval, 2011). Forensic nursing is used to provide care to victims of all ages who have sustained trauma, including those who were victims of intimate partner violence, sexual assault, child maltreatment, elder abuse, human trafficking, strangulation, and trauma (both intentional and nonintentional). The forensic nurse interviews the patient, obtaining information about the person's health history and the crime or trauma to guide his or her assessment. Prior to treating victims, consent is obtained, and the extent of their forensic medical exam and what it can and cannot show is discussed.

This is typically followed by an extensive head-to-toe physical examination for identifying injuries and obtaining forensic evidence that is collected and preserved, maintaining chain of custody. Documentation of injuries is often very detailed, utilizing body maps and diagrams as well as forensic photography when indicated. Injures will often need to be treated after the forensic medical examination. If patients were victims of sexual assaults, they may be affected by sexually transmitted infections, urinary tract infections, infertility issues, vaginal and rectal trauma, and unintended pregnancies that may require treating with prophylactic medications and/or referring patients for further medical treatment and follow-up. Some victims will suffer cardiovascular and respiratory conditions, back pain, dehydration, malnutrition, poor hygiene, or neglect, which can lead to a myriad of medical conditions that may need to be addressed. Lastly, the forensic nurse must resolve any safety issues, implement crisis interventions and advocacy, and file mandatory reports to local reporting agencies.

Fast Facts

A forensic medical examination integrates a head-to-toe assessment and the collection of evidence, which is guided by the forensic interview.

The forensic nurse's responsibilities extend beyond direct patient care and may include duties such as providing education or outreach to the community in which they work. Forensic nurses are the bridge between healthcare and justice and are often called to testify in legal and criminal cases. The forensic nurse is also often involved with larger teams and networks and often interfaces with other medical professionals, law enforcement agencies, criminal justice, victim advocacy, and external agencies that provide additional services to victims.

TYPES OF FORENSIC NURSES AND EDUCATIONAL PREPARATION

Forensic Clinical Nurse Specialist

The forensic clinical nurse specialist is an advanced forensic nursing role that requires a master's or doctoral degree in forensic nursing. Responsibilities of the forensic clinical nurse specialist often include developing and implementing policies relating to various forensic issues and healthcare; conducting research using elements of forensic nursing science; evaluating patient outcomes and engaging in educating others about forensic nursing and evidence-based practices. The forensic clinical nurse specialist may also specialize as a psychiatric forensic nurse, which requires a master's degree in mental health.

Sexual Assault Nurse Examiners

Sexual assault nurse examiners (SANEs) are nurses with additional education, training, and experience in caring for victims of sexual assault. SANE nurses are also trained in addressing victims' medical, psychological, legal, and forensic needs. Currently there are two certifications: one as certified sexual assault nurse examiner for adults (SANE-A) and another as certified sexual assault nurse examiner for pediatrics (SANE-P). The training typically consists of 40 hours of classroom training and then a set number of hours of clinical training under the supervision of a certified SANE and the successful passing of an examination. Maintaining certification includes ongoing education within the specific area, professional activities related to the specific area, and practice hours.

Forensic Nurse Death Investigator

The forensic nurse death investigator was the first recognized type of forensic nursing in the United States (Lynch & Duval, 2011). Each state has its own regulatory laws and policies indicating who can become a death investigator and the requirements for any certification. The American Board of Medicolegal Death Investigators has a certification program that nurses can take to become certified as death investigators.

SCOPE AND STANDARDS OF FORENSIC NURSING PRACTICE

The Scope and Standards of Forensic Nursing Practice (2018) details the core components of forensic nursing. It covers the educational preparation necessary for different forensic nursing roles. Core competencies are highlighted regarding forensic nursing care and how it is delivered.

Examples of competencies of the forensic nurse from the *Scope and Standards of Forensic Nursing Practice* (2018) include the following:

- Collects data of physical and behavioral findings in a systematic and ongoing process with a focus on providing nursing care to patients and for identifying the medicolegal implications of those findings
- Assesses the effect of interactions among individuals, family, community, and social systems on health, illness, safety, and violence and trauma across the life span
- Utilizes complex data and information obtained during interview, examination, diagnostic procedures, and review of medicolegal evidentiary documents in identifying diagnoses
- Defines expected outcomes in terms of the patient, patient's values, ethical considerations, environment, or situation with such considerations as those associated with risks, benefits and costs, medicolegal factors, clinical expertise, and current scientific evidence

INTERNATIONAL ASSOCIATION OF FORENSIC NURSES

The IAFN is the professional nursing association for forensic nurses. It is an international organization and has members from all over the world. Their mission is to enhance the work of forensic nurses by setting standards and fostering the work forensic nurses are doing through developing, promoting, and disseminating information (IAFN, 2018, "Our Mission"). They achieve this through their publications, conferences, educational activities, resources, and member involvement. The IAFN's *Journal of Forensic Nursing* focuses on different aspects of forensic nursing and forensic science and education. The yearly conference meeting hosts various presenters who discuss the latest in forensic science and research. The organization has a member community where forensic nurses from other states and countries can connect and discuss various topics. They have detailed protocols and guidelines for nurses and educational opportunities.

CONCLUSION

Forensic nursing is an ever-growing science that has demonstrated a significant impact on the medical, nursing, and legal systems. Despite a lack of forensic nursing education in entry-level nursing education, nurses working in different sectors will encounter patients for whom forensic nursing skills are used and required. Nurses can stay current on forensic nursing by attending conferences, taking additional continuing education courses, and becoming active members of the forensic nursing community. Until forensic nursing is mandated for all nursing curriculums, nurses should be proactive and seek out educational activities that cover the vast topics of forensic nursing and which patients would benefit from forensic nursing. This will allow nurses to gain insight, knowledge, and skills in caring for patients who would benefit from forensic nursing.

References

Burgess, A. W., & Holmstrom, L. L. (1985). *Rape trauma syndrome and post traumatic stress response. Rape and sexual assault: A research handbook* (pp. 46–60). New York, NY: Garland.

Clark, T. (1976). Counseling victims of rape. *The American Journal of Nursing, 76*(12), 1964–1966. doi:10.1097/00000446-197612000-00024

Galappathie, N., Khan, S. T., & Hussain, A. (2017). Civil and forensic patients in secure psychiatric settings: A comparison. *BJPsych Bulletin, 41*(3), 156–159. doi:10.1192/pb.bp.115.052910

International Association of Forensic Nurses. (n.d.). About us. Retrieved from https://www.forensicnurses.org/page/Overview

International Association of Forensic Nurses. (2018). *Forensic nursing: Scope and standards of practice* (2nd ed.). Elkridge, MD: Author.

Lynch, V., & Duval, J. B. (2011). *Forensic nursing science* (2nd ed.). St. Louis, MO: Mosby/Elsevier.

Maguire, K., & Raso, M. (2017). Reflections on forensic nursing: An interview with Virginia A. Lynch. *Journal of Forensic Nursing, 13*(4), 210–215. doi:10.1097/JFN.0000000000000174

Officer, D. C. (1979). *Healthcare professionals in custody suites—Guidance to supplement revisions to the codes of practice under the Police and Criminal Evidence Act 1984*. Home Office. Drugs Branch, Queen Anne's Gate, London, SW1 9AT. Retrieved from http://webarchive.nationalarchives. gov.uk/20120215212331/http://www.bahamousainquiry.org/linkedfiles/ baha_mousa/module_4/expert_witnesses/jpj/miv008365.pdf

Smith, S. (1951). History and development of forensic medicine. *British Medical Journal, 1*(4707), 599. doi:10.1136/bmj.1.4707.599

Speck, P., & Aiken, M. (1995). 20 years of community nursing service: Memphis Sexual Assault Resource Center. *Tennessee Nurse, 58*(2), 15–18.

2

Medical Examiner Investigator

Meredith J. Scannell

Forensic nurses can take on many different roles, one of which is a medical examiner investigator. Forensic nurses are ideal as medical examiner investigators, utilizing their educational backgrounds in forensics as well as their nursing backgrounds in examining aspects related to death, which may include autopsy, postmortem evidence collection, forensic photography, and interviewing those close to the deceased.

At the end of the chapter, the nurse will be able to:

1. Describe the role and responsibilities of the medical examiner investigator.
2. Understand the complex scenarios where forensic nurses are instrumental as medical examiner investigators.
3. Describe the process in obtaining certification or qualifying as a medical examiner investigator.

BACKGROUND

A medical examiner investigator is someone who investigates the medical and socially relevant circumstances surrounding deaths. Each state has laws and regulations as to who can be a death investigator; in some states nurses are able to work in this role. Nurses who conduct medical examiner death investigations may also be known by different titles: "forensic nurse death investigator" (FNDI), "deputy coroner," or even "coroner." They have the authority to confirm or pronounce death, establish decedent identification, and notify next of kin. Their skills enable them to perform the critical components of death investigation: ascertaining medical and social history of the decedent, examining the body, and investigating the scene. They also work closely with law enforcement, social services, organ and tissue procurement agencies, and the community. A large part of their work is educating families: explaining procedures and test results and interpreting autopsy findings.

Fast Facts

A forensic nurse death investigator role includes the skills and training necessary to investigate death scenes as well as bridging a gap between families and the deceased by education and providing crisis interventions.

COMMON RESPONSIBILITIES OF A MEDICAL EXAMINER INVESTIGATOR

- Respond to scenes of reported deaths
- Determine need for autopsy
- Prepare human remains for transport
- Investigate the circumstances surrounding a death
- Notify next of kin of death
- Issue death certificate
- Pronounce death

The role and scope of practice of the FNDI was largely developed in the early work of Virginia Lynch, who was instrumental in establishing forensic nursing in the United States and the inception of the International Association of Forensic Nurses (IAFN; Lynch, 1989). Working as a FNDI encompasses the scope and practice of nursing. Nurses often have the educational background necessary for death investigations, which includes extensive knowledge in anatomical, medical, and surgical conditions. Nurses also understand and can interpret medical records and documents. In addition, nurses are trained in interview techniques, and they are often empathetic and have therapeutic communication skills that are necessary in dealing with some cases. Additional education, training, or experience in forensic pathology and science make the nurse an ideal candidate for the role of a death investigator (Lynch, 1989).

TRAINING

The role of the FNDI is outlined in IAFN's *Forensic Nursing: Scope and Standards of Practice*. In addition, the IAFN has developed educational guidelines for the forensic nurse death examiner. The training guideline does not elaborate on a certification process; however, it includes detailed information regarding the necessary additional training a nurse would need to become a FNDI (IAFN, 2013).

Training components for FNDI

Forensic nursing science

Multidisciplinary team concepts

Death investigation systems

Roles and responsibilities of FNDI

Evidence management

Criminal justice system

Ethics

Fast Facts

To date there is no specific forensic nursing death investigator course; certification of becoming a death investigator is through the American Board of Medicolegal Death Investigators.

Certification

The American Board of Medicolegal Death Investigators (n.d.) has a certification for individuals who are currently death investigators and have at least 640 hours of death investigations and allows them to apply and sit for an exam that will certify them as death investigators. Other local organizations, colleges, and universities offer fee-based courses in death investigation (Table 2.1).

RESPONSIBILITIES OF A FNDI

When called to a scene, FNDIs must document their findings of the body and its surroundings both in writing and in photographs. They may need to interview witnesses, emergency personnel who arrived first on the scene, fire personnel, as well as hospital staff and those who knew the victim. FNDIs collect evidence from the body and its

Table 2.1

Death Investigator Educational Trainings		
Course	**Description**	**Website**
St. Louis University School of Medicine	Basic medicolegal death investigator training	www.slu.edu/medicine/pathology/medicolegal-deathinvestigators-training
International Association of Coroners and Medical Examiners	Basic and advance death investigation training, annual educational conferences and training symposia	www.theiacme.com
The National Center for Fatality Review and Prevention (national resource and database of child death review teams)	Online webinars and presentations on various topics	www.ncfrp.org

surroundings, knowing what evidence may be pertinent as the investigation progresses. As the representative of the medical examiner's or coroner's office, the FNDI has jurisdiction over the body at a scene and must work in collaboration with the police and other officials involved in the case, obtaining necessary documents and materials that will aid in their investigation. They may also notify the next of kin of the death.

In addition to determining the cause of death, there may also be a need to determine if there was a sexual assault in the context of the death. The process of obtaining samples for sexual assault evidence collection should be done using the local or state evidence collection kit. Additional equipment may be necessary to use during the process, such as a colposcopy, which enhances the visualization of the genital tissue, often allowing for the ability to obtain pictures. Toluidine blue dye may also be used, which is a staining technique that, when applied to injuries or abrasions, will stain the area in a bluish color, allowing for identification of injuries. Throughout the collection of evidence, including body fluids collected during autopsy, the proper chain of custody must be followed for the evidence to be admissible in court, which is the detailed and chronological documentation of the handling of evidence from collection to analysis to disposition. Every transfer of possession of a piece of evidence must be documented.

Forensic nurses who are medical examiners are often chosen for their expertise in grief and ability to provide crisis intervention, which is necessary in some cases of death and death scene investigations (Baumann & Stark, 2015). In some conditions medical death investigations can be difficult, especially in cases of infant deaths. The death scene investigations include close examination of living conditions and interviews of people close to the infant (Cullen, Oberle, Elomba, Stiffler, & Luna, 2016). Questions will be asked about the health of the infant, caregivers, and house and sleeping conditions, and there will be an overall assessment of the immediate living conditions (Cullen, Oberle, Elomba, Stiffler, & Luna, 2016). This may divulge personal details that the family may not want to disclose, such as domestic violence, alcohol misuse, and use of recreational or legal drugs. The situation can turn grim similar to cases of sudden infant death (SID) and unexplained infant death (UIFD), as these are deaths that are unexplained and can cause guilt and suspicious among family members and close contacts. Even if parents or other persons are acquitted of a wrongful death, they will still want answers about the death of the child. This conversation is difficult, as the medical examination shows no determined causes and leaves unanswered questions to an often difficult and sad time. In addition, forensic nurses may be able to provide mementos after the completion of an examination (Cullen, Oberle, Elomba, Stiffler, & Luna, 2016). For parents, this may mean an important connection to their loved baby, such as a footprint or lock of hair, which otherwise may not have been considered and unattainable at the time of death. The National Center for Fatality Review and Prevention is a resource and database for national child death review programs and offers training and educational programs to enhance forensic and death investigation skills.

Medical examiner investigators may also be called upon in cases of mass disasters. FNDIs may play a large role in collecting and preserving evidence, especially in cases where criminal or terrorist activities are involved. They may also assist a disaster mortuary operations team, helping to identify victims or assist local mortuary services.

CONCLUSION

Forensic nurses are qualified in many areas to become medical examiner investigators. They have a fundamental understanding of anatomy, pathophysiology, and various disease processes. With additional education, training, and experience, becoming medical examiner investigators should be a seamless process to advancing their foundational nursing backgrounds. In addition, nurses are skilled in interviewing, developing therapeutic relationships, and dealing with stressful situations, which are key skills in dealing with deaths in which there are complex situations, and may be essential in helping people move from times of crisis and difficulty to times of acceptance and adjustments.

References

American Board of Medicolegal Death Investigators. (n.d.). Registry certification (basic). Retrieved from http://www.abmdi.org/registry_certification

Baumann, R., & Stark, S. (2015). The role of forensic death investigators interacting with the survivors of death by homicide and suicide. *Journal of Forensic Nursing, 11*(1), 28–32. doi:10.1097/JFN.0000000000000058

Cullen, D., Oberle, M., Elomba, C. D., Stiffler, D., & Luna, G. (2016). Illustrations of unexpected infant sleep deaths. *Journal of Forensic Nursing, 12*(3), 141–146. doi:10.1097/JFN.0000000000000120

International Association of Forensic Nurses (IAFN). (2013). *Forensic nurse death investigator education guidelines*. Elkridge, MD: Author. Retrieved from https://www.forensicnurses.org/page/EducationGuidelines

Lynch, V. A. (1989). Forensic nurse examiners. *The American Journal of Nursing, 89*(2), 176. doi:10.2307/3471080

3

Principles of Evidence Collection and Preservation

Meredith J. Scannell

Evidence collection is a key aspect of forensic nursing, which includes the preservation of physical evidence to prevent contamination. It is often done in cases of sexual assault and completed by a sexual assault nurse examiner (SANE). However, SANE nurses are not always available and nurses who work in emergency departments (EDs), intensive care units (ICUs), and operating rooms may need to utilize forensic principles in collecting evidence from various patient populations. Having an understanding of the basic principles limits contamination of evidence and promotes preservation.

At the end of the chapter, the nurse will be able to:

1. Describe the consent process for evidence collection.
2. Describe various components of evidence collection.
3. Identify key aspects in documentation regarding evidence collection.
4. Describe the process for chain of custody.

BACKGROUND

The purpose of a medical forensic exam and subsequent evidence collection is to provide law enforcement with details and evidence that can assist with an investigation. Most often, evidence collection is part of the medical forensic examination of a sexually assaulted patient. The medical forensic examination includes obtaining the patient's consent for the exam, an interview with the patient, documentation of the assault, a physical assessment, and a lengthy evidence collection process. Sexual assault evidence collection kits vary from state to state and should come with directions concerning their contents and perhaps even step-by-step instructions to help guide the individual in what to collect for evidence. There are specific time frames of when evidence should be collected depending upon the time that has passed since the assault, which is most often 120 hours or 5 days. Therefore, it is essential to establish a timeline of when the event occurred and when a patient is seeking treatment. Additionally, some evidence will or will not be collected depending on how much time has lapsed between the assault and when the patient is seeking care. Another consideration is even if the assault occurred more than 5 days ago, the individual may still require immediate care, and depending on the specifics of the assault and injuries, a forensic exam may still be essential to conduct a forensic interview and document injuries.

Fast Facts

The evidence collection process demonstrates only whether trace evidence or someone's DNA profile was or was not present, not that an assault occurred.

CONSENT PROCESS

The first step in a forensic exam is to complete the consent process. All the steps involved and the examination's limitations should be discussed with the patient. The patient should also have an opportunity to ask questions. Patients who are intoxicated at the time of the assault will need to become sober before they can proceed. Evidence should never be collected on an unconscious or impaired patient without legal consent. Any patient who is unable to consent requires a healthcare proxy or, in some cases, a legal consultation. Additionally, many states have mandatory reporting and the healthcare provider is legally obligated to report the incident to the designated organizations. There may also be the issue of the patient's ability to consent to treatment if he or she is a minor. Knowing the state laws on conditions of emancipation is often critical for these patients. A minor may be considered emancipated to make a decision regarding treatment after a sexual assault, but the healthcare provider may still be legally obligated to report the incident to specific state agencies.

Fast Facts

The healthcare provider conducting the exam and obtaining the forensic history should use terminology that the patient understands.

FORENSIC INTERVIEW

After the consent is completed, a forensic interview takes places. Obtaining an accurate forensic history is critical because it guides the healthcare provider when looking for injuries and evidence for collection. Questions should be open-ended, allowing the patient to expand on details. The healthcare professional should refrain from judgment when asking or responding to questions. The written narrative should include the specific details of the assault, preassault activity, postassault activity, and details about the assailant(s). Table 3.1 lists key

Table 3.1

Resources for Forensic Health Practitioners		
Organization	**Type of Resource**	**Web Address**
A National Protocol for Sexual Assault Medical Forensic Examinations Adults/Adolescents	Comprehensive resource manual for healthcare providers in caring for patients who were sexually assaulted	https://www.ncjrs.gov/pdffiles1/ovw/241903.pdf
American College of Emergency Physicians (*Evaluation and management of the sexually assaulted or sexually abused patient,* 2nd ed.)	Comprehensive resource manual for healthcare providers. Includes blank documents and traumagrams	
International Association of Forensic Nurses	International professional organization for forensic nurses. Available resources, education, and information in forensics and certification in becoming a sexual assault nurse examiner	http://www.forensicnurses.org/
BALD STEP Instructions, Carter-Snell, Mount Royal University	Traumagram with instructions and key for documenting injuries	http://www.mtroyal.ca/cs/groups/public/documents/pdf/pdf_baldstepkeyforphysicalfind.pdf

aspects to cover and record in the interview process. This can be a very distressing process and, if available, an advocate or supporting person such as a family member or friend should be present. The forensic interview can be a stressful time for the patient and using a trauma-informed approach is essential to minimize further trauma. Allow the patient to express his or her story and emotions, and allow for a rape crisis advocate to help support the person if there is one available.

BOX 3.1 ITEMS TO CONSIDER FOR A FORENSIC INTERVIEW

- General appearance and demeanor of the patient during visit, that is, tearful, concerned
- Time and location of assault
- Details of assault, sexual acts performed, such as oral, anal, or vaginal penetration; include positions of sexual acts
- Use of verbal or physical coercion
- Types of weapon, force, hitting, chocking, restraints, burns used during the assault
- Objects used during the assault
- Other nongenital acts, kissing, touching, licking, biting, and where on the body
- Use of condoms, or lubricants, and information regarding if and where ejaculation occurred
- Pain, injuries, or bleeding that has occurred
- Use of alcohol or drugs
- Alterations in memory or consciousness
- The transfer of bodily fluids
- Use of foreign bodies or objects
- Assailant(s) (note brief description only)
- Relationship to assailant, that is, stranger, acquaintance, Internet connection

Fast Facts

When documenting a forensic interview, it is critical to differentiate whether penetration occurred, even if it was slight, as this is the legal difference between rape and indecent assault.

CONTROL SWABS

Control swabs may be used as a standard. These swabs are moistened with sterile water and used for the entire evidence collection process.

Fast Facts

Wear gloves when collecting evidence and change them on a regular basis or between different samples of evidence collection so that cross-contamination does not occur.

VICTIM'S DNA

Part of the evidence collection process is also obtaining the victim's DNA, commonly by obtaining a blood or buccal sample. A buccal sample is obtained with large swabs taken from the inside of the victim's cheek.

ORAL EVIDENCE COLLECTION

If there was an oral assault, then evidence should be collected within the time frame allowed. Most often, this is 24 hours, as the likelihood of evidence beyond that point is low. Prior to swabbing, there should be an assessment of the mouth for any injuries. The use of an alternative light source may also be helpful in identifying possible substances that should be swabbed. For oral evidence, swab between the lips, teeth, and gums and rotate the swabs during collection.

FINGERNAIL SCRAPING SAMPLES

Fingernail scrapings should be collected as per protocol. For evidence collection kits that contain this step, this will be performed on most patients. Using a nail scraper, scrape nail debris from each hand over a piece of paper and then collect the contents as well as the scraper for evidence collection. In cases where the patient has short fingernails, moist swabs can be used on the fingernail areas.

HEAD HAIR SAMPLES

Obtaining head hair samples should be done as per protocol. This most often includes a small comb and piece of paper; the hair is combed over the paper so that any loose hair or debris falls onto the paper. The comb and paper are collected for analysis. For patients with hair difficult to comb, lightly run the comb over the hair or have the patient shake their hair vigorously over the paper to cause loose hair and debris to fall.

BITE MARKS

Bite marks will also need to be swabbed and measured. The best place to obtain evidence is where the lips would have touched the skin around the bite. Use moistened swabs on the area where the teeth and lips of the assailant would have pressed on the patient's skin. Document the bite mark on an anatomical drawing or traumagram and include a detailed description and measurements.

PUBIC HAIR COMBINGS

If patients have pubic hair, this may need to be collected. In cases where the patient has no or minimal pubic hair, moistened swabs can be used on the area to collect evidence.

Fast Facts

Several evidence collection swabs may be necessary for the pubic area. Having the equipment ready will help expedite the process and limit any unnecessary exposure to the patient.

VAGINAL EVIDENCE

If there was a vaginal assault, then evidence should be collected in the vagina. Unlike the oral and rectal areas, semen can be present in the vagina up to 5 days after an assault. The vaginal area may require several swabs for evidence collection. When first examining the area, start with the inner thighs and pubic areas and check for any injuries, contusions, or areas with which the assailant may have come in contact. Next, the external vagina should be inspected for trauma, or areas where semen may have dried. An alternative light source may be used. Any area that fluoresces under the florescent light should be swabbed with moistened swabs and documented on the traumagram. For the internal vaginal evidence, a speculum is moistened with sterile water and inserted into the vagina. First, the vaginal vault should be inspected for any foreign bodies and then inspected for injuries. The cervix should be examined for any injuries, abrasions, and bruising as well as the possible presence of a sexually transmitted infection, which would appear as a purulent discharge from the cervix. A specimen should be collected by swabbing the posterior fornix below the cervix where semen may have pooled. A moistened swab is not necessary, as the area inside the vagina is already moist. All evidence findings should be documented and any foreign bodies should be collected and dried for evidence.

PERINEAL EVIDENCE

Swabbing the perineal area is required if there was a rectal or vaginal assault. The area should first be inspected for any injuries and swabbed with moistened swabs.

PENILE EVIDENCE

Penile swabs are taken when there was an assault to the penis. Using swabs moistened with distilled water, swab the glands, shaft, and base of the penis with a rotating motion to ensure uniform sampling.

Fast Facts

For some patients swabbing the penis can be uncomfortable. One approach to obtaining these swabs is to instruct the patients on how they can do the penile swabs themselves. This allows them to actively participate in the process and makes them more comfortable.

RECTAL EVIDENCE

If there was a rectal assault, then swabs should be taken in under 24 hours. Examine the buttocks and perianal skin for signs of injury. The area should first be assessed for injury, using gentle separation of the perianal skin to inspect the anal verge for signs of lacerations or abrasions. When taking an anorectal swab and smear, moisten the swabs and swab the area first for the smear slides and then repeat the procedure with the second set of swabs.

FOREIGN MATERIAL

A thorough inspection for any foreign material on the patient's body should be completed and any findings collected for evidence. Patients should undress over a large piece of paper or sheet in case any loose debris falls so it can then be collected. Loose debris that should be collected can include leaves, grass, or loose hair that may not be the patient's. Any loose debris or foreign material should be placed in the center of a piece of paper or sheet and then folded in a manner that keeps the material within the paper or sheet. Often, material is found within the vagina and should be dried if wet. However, certain material may require additional drying time. If a tampon needs to be collected and it is not possible to air-dry it completely, place the tampon in a urine specimen container and puncture some holes in the lid. This will allow the tampon to be dried and preserved. Some patients may have also been brought in by ambulance on a bed sheet; this too can be collected for evidence as it may contain debris that fell off the patient and may be valuable in establishing where the crime occurred, especially if there are specific rug fibers that can be traced or dirt specific to the crime scene.

CLOTHING COLLECTION

There are times when clothing from the victim needs to be collected. It is recommended that underwear is always collected, even several days after the assault, as fluids that may have leaked out of the vaginal vault could contain semen. All clothing items should be separately collected and documented and then placed in a larger collection transportation bag with the chain of custody form enclosed. It is important to find out the policy regarding patients getting their clothing back; in some cases, they may not get their clothing back and some may not want to have a clothing item included in the evidence collection kit. It is extremely important not to cut through any existing holes, rips, or stains, as they may indicate other evidence, such as a hole from a gunshot wound, and it may be essential to maintain its integrity.

ADDITIONAL SWABS

Swab any area when the patient indicates it relates to the history or suspicion of bodily fluid transfer, such as licking, kissing, or biting, or areas where there may be other trace evidence. An alternative light source, such as the wood lamp, will help identify possible areas that need to be swabbed. It is best to have the patient undress, and then turn off the lights and examine the patient's body to see if any areas indicate the need for a swab. There may also be circumstances where you need to swab objects. For example, if a patient was wearing a valuable ring and blood or semen may have touched it, this object can be swabbed.

TOXICOLOGY TESTING

In some circumstances, it may be necessary to obtain toxicology testing when there was a suspected drug-facilitated assault. Signs include memory loss, unconsciousness, drowsiness, abnormal loss of inhibition, or a discrepancy in the amount of alcohol consumed and behavior, or if the patient believes they may have been drugged or given something. It is critical that the patient is notified that the toxicology test will assess the presence of substances, such as drugs and alcohol, both legal and illegal. There is often a time limit on performing toxicology testing, which is around 96 hours since the time of the assault or the time during which substances were believed to be ingested.

INJURY DOCUMENTATION

It is critical to document injuries accurately and thoroughly, even if photographs have been taken. A body diagram map should be used for documenting injuries and foreign bodies to demonstrate where they occurred on the body, including the size, depth, shape, and pattern of the injury and measurements if possible. All injuries or bruises should be measured and documented with a standard technique. The BALD STEP mnemonic focuses on trauma-related injuries and allows for more precise documentation of general and genital injuries as well as documenting cases of strangulation. The acronym stands for the following injury types.

B: bite mark, bleeding, bruise, burn

A: abrasion, avulsion

L: laceration

D: deformity

S: swelling, stains

T: tenderness, trace evidence

E: erythema

P: patterns, petechiae, penetrating wounds

Vaginal injuries can be common in cases of sexual assault and the use of other techniques has been implemented in assisting with injury identification. The most common area of genital injuries is in the posterior fourchette, around the six o'clock position, and the labia minora. The use of staining helps to visualize injuries that are difficult to detect otherwise. Toluidine blue dye 1% stains injuries, lacerations, and abrasions blue. A colposcopy has the benefits of magnifying and photographing the area; however, this equipment may not be readily available. Using either toluidine blue dye or a colposcopy typically results in higher rates of injuries being found when compared to an examination with the naked eye. Regardless of method, assessment of genital injuries should always precede a speculum or pelvic examination as injuries can result from these exams.

PHOTO DOCUMENTATION

It may be necessary to obtain photo documentation. Forensic photos require a strict process. Different states, hospitals, and healthcare centers may have policies on photo documentation and these should guide the practice. Fundamental aspects should, however, be followed. All injuries should have a close and long-range photo with a measurement included, such as a ruler. If a ruler or measurement tool is unavailable, then a standard object such as a coin should be included in the pictures to allow for accurate measurements. In some jurisdiction, photographs of the genital areas are not recommended and injuries in these areas should be documented on a traumagram. When taking photographs, it is also important to pay attention to the background and have the patient in an area that limits unnecessary background items in the photo. The patient's face should be neutral, and the patient's privacy should be maintained with parts of the body covered up that do not require being photographed. Patient confidentiality and the Health Insurance Portability and Accountability Act (HIPAA) practices should be adhered to when taking and storing documents in medical or electronic records.

CHAIN OF CUSTODY

The chain of custody is an essential aspect of the evidence collection process. Once evidence collection begins, the individual collecting the evidence must maintain a chain of custody and needs to maintain possession of the collected evidence until it is signed, sealed, and locked in a refrigerator for collection by law enforcement. This ensures the kit's integrity, which may otherwise come into question during legal proceedings.

CONCLUSION

Evidence collection can be an extremely stressful time for the patient and even the healthcare professional who is conducting the evidence collection. Having open and honest communication with the patient will help. Inform him or her that you need to follow the directions and need to take your time so that the evidence collected is complete. Allow the patient to take his or her time, and if evidence collection is too stressful for the patient, then some steps may need to be skipped over in efforts not to further traumatize the patient. Approaching evidence collection in an empathetic manner will allow you to obtain necessary evidence without traumatizing the patient, which is the ultimate guiding principle.

References

American College of Emergency Physicians. (2013) *Evaluation and management of the sexually assaulted or sexually abused patient* (2nd ed.). Irving, TX: American College of Emergency Physicians.

Burg, A., Kahn, R., & Welch, K. (2011). DNA testing of sexual assault evidence: The laboratory perspective. *Journal of Forensic Nursing, 7*(3), 145–152. doi:10.1111/j.1939-3938.2011.01111.x

Carter-Snell, C. (2011). Injury documentation: Using the BALD STEP mnemonic and the RCMP sexual assault kit. *Outlook, 34*(1), 15–20. https://www.researchgate.net/profile/Catherine_Carter-Snell/publication/225298479_Injury_documentation_Using_the_BALD_STEP_mnemonic_and_the_RCMP_Sexual_Assault_Kit/links/0912f4fd8d450a47f0000000/Injury-documentation-Using-the-BALD-STEP-mnemonic-and-the-RCMP-Sexual-Assault-Kit.pdf

Henry, T. (2013). *Atlas of sexual violence.* St. Louis, MO: Elsevier Mosby.

Ingemann-Hansen, O., & Charles, A. V. (2013). Forensic medical examination of adolescent and adult victims of sexual violence. *Best Practice & Research Clinical Obstetrics & Gynaecology, 27*(1), 91–102. doi:10.1016/j.bpobgyn.2012.08.014

Sachs, C. J., Weinberg, E., & Wheeler, M. W. (2008). Sexual assault nurse examiners' application of statutory rape reporting laws. *Journal of Emergency Nursing, 34*(5), 410–413. doi:10.1016/j.jen.2008.02.010

Scannell, M., MacDonald, A. E., & Foster, C. (2017). Strangulation: What every nurse must recognize. *Nursing Made Incredibly Easy, 15*(6), 41–46. doi:10.1097/01.NME.0000525552.06539.02

U.S. Department of Justice, Office on Violence Against Women. (2013). *A national protocol for sexual assault medical forensic examinations: Adults/adolescents* (2nd ed.). Washington, DC: Author.

4

Providing Testimony in Forensic Cases

Barbara P. Madden

Evidence shows that forensic nurses make a difference in court cases. Sexual assault nurse examiner (SANE) programs and SANE certifications were developed with the aim of providing excellent care for sexual assault patients and improving the quality of evidence in cases that went forward into the court system. From the legal aspect, there are three perspectives to be examined. First, quality assurance programs by crime laboratories indicate that sexual assault kits are more complete and follow legal guidelines for documentation and chain of custody more closely when done by SANEs than those done by non-SANEs. Second, SANEs are better prepared for an encounter with the legal system and testifying in court through their education than either non-SANEs or other emergency room personnel. Third, the literature suggests that the existence of SANE programs in a community can contribute to increased prosecution rates for sexual crimes (Campbell, Greeson, & Patterson, 2011).

At the end of the chapter, the nurse will be able to:

1. Understand the different roles of the forensic nurse as an expert witness versus a fact witness.
2. Become familiar with the preparation necessary for testifying in a forensic case.

3. Follow effective court demeanor and tips for testifying.
4. Perform appropriate evaluation of the forensic nurse's performance in trials.

There are two types of witness categories in which a forensic nurse may be involved: expert witness and percipient witness. Both types of witness have different roles and expectations and often differ by employment.

EXPERT WITNESSES

Being an expert nurse is not the same as being an expert witness. An expert witness is called to testify to the underlying scientific rationale, the validity of procedures used, and their applicability to the facts of the case. It is testimony about what should have been done in the case, not about what the nurse actually did or the facts duly documented. An expert nurse witness has expertise within his or her specific nursing role and can give an expert opinion or draw conclusions on a specific topic or area. They are often asked to testify in cases of malpractice or in cases where there is a disciplinary hearing against another healthcare professional, since they can give a professional opinion on the actions of others. Expert nurse witnesses are often sought after by attorneys and may advertise their services accordingly.

The Daubert standard, first articulated by the courts in 1993, is a rule of evidence regarding the admissibility of expert witnesses' testimonies. Either prosecution or defense may raise a Daubert special motion before or during trial to exclude unqualified evidence being presented to the jury (US Legal, n.d.). A recent example of this is a two-part article in *The New York Times Magazine* (Colloff, 2018a, 2018b) regarding admissibility of testimony on blood spatter analysis, in which the "expert witness" had minimal educational and experiential credentials. The forensic nurse who serves as an expert witness is held to higher standards of relevant education and experience than the nurse testifying about the care provided to a specific forensic patient. Be aware also that, at least in theory, a forensic nurse expert witness may be called by the defense to critique the procedures or counteract the testimony of a percipient nurse witness.

Another type of expert nurse who may become an expert witness is one who becomes a legal nurse consultant and undergoes an additional educational and certification process. Certification of a legal nurse consultant is through the Legal Nurse Consulting Certification Board, which recognizes a nurse's knowledge, skills, and expertise. Legal nurse consultants provide consultation and expertise on a specific topic

(American Association of Legal Nurse Consultants, n.d.). They are trained in conducting a comprehensive analysis and evaluation of specific facts, documents, and testimony and are able to translate that into an expert opinion. They may work alongside attorneys in providing an expert nursing opinion or guidance in certain cases or may testify in actual courtrooms regarding their expert opinions. They may work for insurance companies, pharmaceutical agencies, hospitals, legal firms, governmental agencies, and independent consultation firms.

PERCIPIENT WITNESSES

While there may be instances where forensic nurses are called on to serve as "expert" witnesses, the much more common court experiences are as "percipient" or "fact" witnesses. This occurs when a nurse in the course of practice is in possession of facts, direct observations, and/or personal knowledge of the case at trial. The nurse can testify to physical findings such as lab results, photographs or anatomical drawings, direct observations of behaviors, specimen collection procedures, instruments used to examine clients, and recommendations made regarding treatment and referrals. He or she cannot draw conclusions as can an expert witness and, in many cases, cannot directly testify to "hearsay" regarding patients' statements unless it is as a "fresh complaint" witness (i.e., the very first to hear their story). The vast majority of forensic cases will fall under state jurisdiction, and state laws may differ in terms of what will or will not be allowed as testimony from the forensic nurse. Cases may fall under a variety of jurisdictions:

- Federal Court—examples include immigration issues or interstate issues
- State Superior Court—most felonies; rapes fall under the category of felony
- District Court—most misdemeanors

Fast Facts

Most hospitals and free-standing clinics have (or should have) a specific cart for use in sexual assault forensic exams. All nurses in these settings should be familiar with its contents and which staff member is accountable for appropriate stocking of supplies. Most important is availability of the so-called "rape" kit that contains the documentation forms that will be used in testimony.

- Criminal Court—cases where conviction results in jail time and a criminal record; sexual assaults are dealt with in a criminal court
- Civil Court—cases where a conviction results in fines (to the state) or restitution (to plaintiffs or their estates)
- Juvenile Court—defendants under 17 years of age (if a felony, can be transferred to an adult court)
- Appeals Court—appeals made on the basis of errors of legal procedure, not of factual testimony, unlikely to include forensic nurse testimony

The majority of cases with which a forensic nurse witness will deal will likely fall under Superior Court, Criminal Court, or possibly Juvenile Court.

CASE STUDY

A young woman came to the emergency room complaining of being sexually assaulted. She had been walking to public transportation on her way to work when a stranger driving by offered her a lift to the station. She had mild symptoms of cerebral palsy and the weather was bad; he was young, clean-cut, and had a child seat in the rear of the car, so she decided to accept. Instead, he drove her to an isolated area, pushed her seat back, pulled her slacks and panties down while restraining her with his body weight, and vaginally penetrated her. He then dropped her off at the station where she approached the transit police. She was able to give a partial license plate number and car description as well as a fairly good description of the assailant himself. During the police investigation, two other similarly described cases were noted from the same area: one a young teenager and the second a young woman on crutches. There were two or three other sexual assault kits with similar elements but these unfortunately were unreported cases. The likely assailant was identified but fled the country before trial. Three years later, he was apprehended in his own country, extradited, and returned for prosecution. Three different SANEs for the three reported cases were called to testify at his trial.

PLANNING FOR TESTIFYING BEGINS LONG BEFORE THE ACTUAL TRIAL

- The nurse's professional resume should be current, since it will be required by the prosecutor and defense attorney and will be referenced in testimony to indicate basic credentials as well as specific training and continuing education in the forensic specialty. Certification as a SANE-A, SANE-P, or forensic nurse specialist by the International Association of Forensic Nurses (IAFN)/American Nurses Association (ANA) is desirable. Other forensic credentials are also available. *All three SANEs involved were certified as SANE-Adult and Adolescent by the Commonwealth of Massachusetts* (ANA, 2018; IAFN, 2018).

- Early discussion with the prosecutor is essential to determine the overall legal strategy, what questions might be asked, and likely tactics of the defense. The forensic nurse can suggest areas for questioning or demonstrative evidence that might be introduced. Differences in states' legal processes should also be clarified. *All three SANEs met with the prosecutor to review their testimony. In the above case study, an unusual occurrence was that the defendant served as his own attorney, giving opening statements, questioning witnesses (including the victims!), and providing summation. The court required him to have a public defender sitting with him during the trial to prevent errors leading to a mistrial.* Another possible variant is the defendant's choice of either a jury or a "bench" trial where the judge decides the verdict. *This defendant chose a jury trial.*

- Case preparation should include, at a minimum, a review of the case documentation, relevant current literature and research, nursing and/or specialty standards of care (ANA, 2015, 2017), the state's nurse practice act, and policies and procedures of the nurse's employing agency or contract. If paperwork regarding the patient encounter is not directly available through the SANE's employment protocols, the documentation will have been subpoenaed by the prosecutor and should be provided to the SANE prior to court appearance. *The case study represents a 3-year delay between nursing care provided and actual trial. This is not unusual and highlights the need for careful review of documentation, which was provided by the prosecutor to all three SANEs, and any changes in prescribed procedures between the two time periods.*

Fast Facts

Nurses conducting forensic examinations must be acutely aware of trauma-informed research that may impact on both the patient presentation in the initial care setting and also in the courtroom. Nurses must be prepared to explain posttraumatic stress disorder (PTSD) and its neurobiological manifestations.

IMMEDIATE TRIAL PREPARATION

- Witness demeanor is important; first impressions count, particularly with juries. Relaxation techniques are helpful, but humor is inappropriate. Neither informal scrubs nor extremely formal wear is appropriate. Business casual is a happy medium, and jewelry, hair (including facial), and makeup should be restrained. Professional confidence, but not arrogance, should be portrayed, in articulateness and body language.

- Nurses' testimony should convey impartiality; their role represents the search for truth, not a "win" for the victim (or defendant). They are present to be objective witnesses of the facts and the science base, contributing information to the jury and court so that the most informed disposition of the case can be made. This includes demeanor in the courthouse and outside of the actual courtroom. Excessive friendliness with the prosecutor, law enforcement, or even the victim where you might be observed by the jurors or court officials can damage your credibility.

- Assertive patient advocacy is appropriate in the clinical setting, but not in a court of law. Nurses should never testify that they believe the victim is telling the truth about being assaulted or whether the victim consented to sexual behavior; that is for the jury to decide. It is interesting to note that there is evidence that SANE programs with a strong prosecutorial orientation have greater nurse burnout and vicarious trauma when compared with those with a strong patient care orientation (Campbell, Greeson, & Patterson, 2011).

- When testifying, never "guess" an answer. If you do not know, say so clearly. If it would help to refer to your documentation, ask the judge for permission to do so. If it is necessary to think about your answer, take the time to do so. Be accurate and consistent in your answers, not only in the current trial but across other trials in which you might have testified.

- Understanding the jury's mentality is vital to connecting with them. Scientific evidence is frequently beyond the average juror's

Fast Facts

SANE nurses and others who regularly interact with legal, police, or other justice system personnel need to have an administrative system backup to clearly delineate the different roles each play in justice prosecution, to prevent the perception (or reality) of bias for or against alleged assailants or victims.

understanding. One role of the forensic nurse is juror education in the science behind his or her testimony. Counteract the crime scene investigation (CSI) effect, that is, that all new technology must be used, that DNA must be available in every case, and that immediate (10 minutes on TV) analysis is not standard. Eye contact with jurors is important.

■ The nurse must also realize that juror selection can be manipulated by both prosecutors and defense attorneys, to the perceived advantage of either side. This is accomplished by juror challenges for cause (unlimited) or peremptory challenges (a limited number of challenges that do not need a rationale).

CONDUCT OF A TRIAL

The forensic nurse, as a witness in a trial, is usually not permitted to hear other witnesses' testimonies, so it is useful to know the usual sequence of events that occur in the courtroom in the nurse witness' absence.

■ The assistant district attorney (ADA) may present opening arguments, which are generally a statement of what they intend to prove.
■ The defense attorneys may present similar arguments regarding what they intend to disprove.
■ The ADA presents and questions the prosecution witnesses ("direct"), usually including the victim.
■ After each prosecution witness testifies, the defense attorney may cross-examine him or her.
■ The defense attorney presents and questions the defense witnesses and possibly the defendant ("direct").
■ The ADA may cross-examine the defense witnesses and defendant after each testifies.
■ There may or may not be re-direct and re-cross examinations.
■ The ADA presents closing arguments and summation.
■ The defense attorney presents closing arguments and summation.
■ The case goes to the jury or judge for a decision. Occasionally, there may be a "hung jury" in which no unanimous decision occurs. The prosecution then decides whether to retry the case.
■ If the decision goes against the defendant, sentencing is pronounced. This is often after a period of time, not directly after the decision. The prosecutor and defense attorney may make recommendations regarding the sentence, and a victim impact statement may be allowed.

ACTUAL TESTIMONY: TIPS FOR FORENSIC NURSE WITNESSES

- Be prepared to speak to the jurors directly, using nontechnical terms whenever possible.
- Pause briefly after a question is asked to assure no objection is raised. *This was particularly important in the noted case, since some questions came from an untrained "defense attorney."*
- Respond directly to the jury (or judge in a bench trial), not to the questioning attorney.
- Answer *only* the question asked. Make sure there is only one question asked at a time. Do not respond to the "Don't you agree that . . ." type question, which is frequently complex and not subject to a single or simple answer and a ploy used by the defense. Ask for a breakdown of each question element.
- Some courts permit juries to ask questions of witnesses. Wait for the judge to permit this or to deem it appropriate for your area of expertise.
- Realize that the courtroom is by definition an adversarial system. Extensive cross-examination by the opposing side is standard and should not to be perceived as a personal attack on the nurse as a professional or forensic nurse, but rather the legal duty of the attorney to provide the best possible defense for the client. This cross-examination may be disparagement of a nurse's credentials or experience, or may challenge the accuracy of documentation or the following of procedures or, indeed, anything else the witness might say. *In the case study, nursing credentials were not challenged, but the defendant attempted to malign the integrity of the chain of custody procedures by questioning the witness as to whether proper procedure was followed and opining how the police could have inserted the defendant's DNA into the kit between the time the SANE sealed it and the time of laboratory processing* (Markowitz, 2017).

BOX 4.1 SAMPLE QUESTIONS THAT MAY BE ASKED

Regarding Your Background

- What is your educational background?
- Where are you currently employed?
- What is a SANE nurse?

Regarding the Case

- When you conducted the evidence collection on the patient, did you follow the directions in the order recommended? If not, why not?

(continued)

BOX 4.1 SAMPLE QUESTIONS THAT MAY BE ASKED (*continued*)

Regarding Your Background

- What training was involved in obtaining that designation?
- Is there continuing education required for maintaining your SANE credentials?
- How long have you been working in your role as a SANE?
- Approximately how many evidence collection kits have you conducted?
- How long does it take you to do a typical examination and evidence collection?

Regarding the Case

- Did the patient consent to the exam?
- Explain what you mean by the "demeanor" of the patient.
- Who wrote the narrative and how is that process carried out?
- Explain the terminology you used on the "body map."
- What follow-up did you recommend to the patient after the evidence collection was complete?

COURT RESULT IN THE CASE STUDY

All three SANEs followed the above restrictions on practice/testimony. The defendant was sentenced to 15 years in prison and faced likely deportation at their conclusion. The three victims were vindicated, obtaining a measure of closure despite their ordeal of having to answer questions from their assailant.

POSTTESTIMONY QUALITY IMPROVEMENT/EVALUATION

- It is often helpful to have an objective colleague in the courtroom to provide feedback on your testimony and how it was received/ perceived. You as the witness may not be able to process juror reactions, but a friend may.
- You can also contact the prosecutor (ADA) for recommendations on performance improvement. Specifically ask about comments by the opposing attorney, jury, or judge about your testimony, such as in closing arguments, instructions to the jury, or postpolling of jurors. Witnesses are not able to view these proceedings themselves.
- No court result is likely to be ideal from all perspectives. Do not judge the quality of your witness "performance" by the verdict.

It is tempting to despair or self-blame if your testimony did not result in a conviction that you fully expected; realize that many factors other than your individual testimony enter into a jury's decision.

CONCLUSION

While the notion of testifying in a court case that might be traumatic for your sexual assault patient and/or life-damaging for the alleged assailant is a daunting one, nurses have conquered similar hurdles many times in their professional lives. Familiarity with the legal processes, meticulous preparation for testifying on the stand, and an excellent grounding in standards of ethical professional practice are the keys to competent performance as a nurse/forensic witness.

References

American Association of Legal Nurse Consultants. (n.d.). What is an LNC? Retrieved from http://www.aalnc.org/page/what-is-an-lnc

American Nurses Association. (2015). *Nursing: Scope and standards of practice* (3rd ed.). Silver Spring, MD: Author.

American Nurses Association. (2018). *Advanced forensic nursing (AFN-BC)*. Silver Spring, MD: Author.

American Nurses Association and International Association of Forensic Nurses. (2017). *Forensic nursing: Scope and standards of practice* (2nd ed.). Silver Spring, MD: Authors.

Campbell, R., Greeson, M., & Patterson, D. (2011). Defining the boundaries: How sexual assault nurse examiners (SANEs) balance patient care and law enforcement collaboration. *Journal of Forensic Nursing, 7*, 17–26. doi:10.1111/j.1939-3938.2010.01091.x

Colloff, P. (2018a, May 23). Blood will tell: Part 1. *New York Times Magazine*. Retrieved from https://www.nytimes.com/interactive/2018/05/23/magazine/joe-bryan-blood-forensics-murder.html

Colloff, P. (2018b, May 31). Blood will tell: Part 2. *New York Times Magazine*. Retrieved from https://www.nytimes.com/interactive/2018/05/31/magazine/joe-bryan-part-2-blood-spatter-analysis-faulty-evidence.html

International Association of Forensic Nurses (IAFN). (2018). *SANE-A and SANE-P certifications*. Elkridge, MD: IAFN.

Markowitz, J. (2017, October 12). *Evaluating the treating clinician's testimony: A defense expert's perspective*. Presentation at the International Conference on Forensic Nursing Science and Practice Annual Conference, Toronto, ON, Canada.

US Legal. (n.d.). Daubert challenge law and legal definitions. Retrieved from https://definitions.uslegal.com/d/daubert-challenge

5

Trauma-Informed Care:
Treating the Whole Person

Diane L. Miller

Trauma has lasting adverse effects on a person's physical, psychological, social, and spiritual well-being. It affects every aspect of a person's life, including physical health, behavioral health, the ability to learn, as well as relationships. The earlier in life the trauma occurs, the more damaging the consequences may be (Blanche, 2012; Machtinger et al., 2015; Reeves & Humphreys, 2017; Stokes et al., 2017). As forensic nurses, we recognize that trauma survivors are vulnerable and that we must provide culturally competent, gender-neutral, recovery-oriented care.

Trauma-informed care (TIC) means treating the whole person while considering and attempting to understand past traumatic events and how they may influence current behaviors and coping mechanisms. We must consider the complexities of a person's lived experiences as integral to the decisions and choices that the person makes.

TIC helps us to "see" the bigger picture. It will help us to understand that victims of traumatic events will not always react or behave in ways we expect. It is often said that traumatic reactions are normal reactions to abnormal situations (Withers, 2017).

At the end of the chapter, the nurse will be able to:

1. Discuss how pervasive trauma is in our society and the impact it has on public health.
2. Recognize the importance of understanding the trauma patient's past lived experiences when providing nursing care to the victim of a current traumatic event.
3. Integrate forensic nursing practice into the core principles of TIC to empower patients to participate in their healthcare decisions.

TRAUMA

The American Psychological Association (2018) describes "trauma" as exposure to actual or threatened death, serious injury, or violence. Trauma is an emotional response to a terrible life event in the life story of a patient who has directly experienced an event such as childhood or adult physical, sexual, or emotional abuse; neglect; loss; community violence; structural violence; or terrorism. Trauma also encompasses the life stories of our patients who have personally witnessed an event occurring to others or learned that such an event happened to a close family member or friend.

Trauma is our life story—the care providers who note repeated or extreme exposure to aversive details of such events.

TRAUMA-INFORMED CARE

TIC recognizes the impact of interpersonal violence and victimization on an individual's life and development (Reeves & Humphreys, 2017; Stokes et al., 2017). To provide TIC, we must seek to understand how violence impacts the lives of patients and be aware that every interaction we have with patients is consistent with the recovery process and reduces the possibility of retraumatization by the care we provide.

BOX 5.1 TRAUMA IS AN EMOTIONAL RESPONSE TO A TERRIBLE EVENT

- Trauma and its consequences are recognized as serious public health risks.
- Most mental health professionals do not have formal education and training in trauma mental health.
- Trauma affects up to 60% of the American population.

Trauma survivors are the majority of patients in human service systems and we must recognize we have no way of distinguishing survivors from nonsurvivors. To provide TIC means we treat all patients as if they were survivors by implementing strategies to reduce retraumatization and recognizing that the effects of trauma can be seen in the problems directly or indirectly related to the trauma (Blanche, 2012; Bowen & Murshid, 2016; Reeves & Humphreys, 2017; Stokes et al., 2017).

TIC: A STRENGTH-BASED FRAMEWORK

Trauma symptoms arising from past violence and the absence of a safe environment create obstacles to services, treatment, and recovery. TIC recognizes that the violence of trauma is both physical and psychological in nature. Concentrate your care on what has happened to the person, not on his or her response to the trauma. TIC provides "do no harm" care and does not retraumatize or blame victims for trying to manage their traumatic reactions to abnormal situations (Reeves & Humphreys, 2017). Nurses must remember that the person may be experiencing thoughts, feelings, or behaviors that remind him or her of past traumatic events, thus precipitating a stress response even if the person is now in a safe place.

Fast Facts

TIC shifts our focus to "What happened to you?"

Trauma affects all genders, all ages, known survivors, and new survivors; trauma is acute and chronic.

TIC is a powerful framework: It gives hope and a new culture to provide a better way to handle trauma, which is one of our most pressing social issues (Blanche, 2012; Bowen & Murshid, 2016). The core principles of providing TIC are essential to the work and care forensic nurses deliver (Table 5.1). TIC guides how we approach, know, and treat our patients.

EMPOWERING OUR PATIENTS

The prevalence of trauma in the United States is sobering:

- One in four women experience intimate partner violence.
  - One in four women experience severe physical violence.
  - About 8.5 million women experience rape before the age of 18.

Table 5.1

Core Principles of TIC	
Core Principle	**Approach**
Safety	Provide physical and emotional safety.
	Prevent further trauma from occurring.
Trustworthiness and transparency	Maintain transparency in policy and procedure.
	Build trust among staff, patients, and community members.
Collaboration and peer support	View patients as central members of the care team and experts in their own lives.
	Operationalize peer support and peer mentoring.
Empowerment and choice	Share power with patients; give them a strong voice in decision making.
Minimization of retraumatization	Recognize the potential for retraumatization.
	Understand the impact of trauma and how the current problem may relate.
	Protect the patient from any power differential.
	Recognize the patient's fears and expectations.

TIC, trauma-informed care.

Source: Blanch, A. (2012). *SAMHSA'S National Center for Trauma Informed Care: Changing communities, changing lives: Substance abuse and mental health services administration.* Rockville, MD: Substance Abuse and Mental Health Services Administration. Retrieved from https://www.nasmhpd.org/sites/default/files/NCTIC_Marketing_Brochure_FINAL(2).pdf; Bowen, E. A., & Murshid, S. M. (2016). Trauma-informed social policy: A conceptual framework for policy analysis and advocacy. *Perspectives from the Social Sciences, 106*(2), 223–229. doi:10.2105/AJPH.2015.302970; Machtinger, E. L., Cuca, Y. P., Khanna, N., Rose, C. D., & Kimberg, L. S. (2015). From treatment to healing: The promise of trauma-informed primary care. *Women's Health Issues, 25*(3), 193–197. doi:10.1016/j .whi.2015.03.008; Reeves, E. A., & Humphreys, J. C. (2017). Describing the healthcare experiences and strategies of women survivors of violence. *Journal of Clinical Nursing, 27,* 1170–1182. doi:10.1111/jocn.14152; Stokes, Y., Jacob, J. D., Gifford, W., Squires, J., & Vandyk, A. (2017). Exploring nurses' knowledge and experiences related to traumainformed care. *Global Qualitative Nursing Research, 4,* 1–10. doi:10 .1177/2333393617734510

- One in nine men experience intimate partner violence.
  - One in seven men experience severe physical violence.
  - About 1.5 million men were made to penetrate before the age of 18.
- One in four children experience maltreatment (physical, sexual, or emotional abuse).
  - About 1,640 children died from child maltreatment in 2012 (CDC, 2014, 2017).

BOX 5.2 TRAUMATIC REACTIONS: NORMAL REACTIONS TO ABNORMAL SITUATIONS

Prolonged and repeated episodes of childhood and adult trauma can lead to complex posttraumatic stress disorder (PTSD), which can have prolonged effects on emotional regulation, self-perception, and relationships with others. This helps to explain many of the reactions and coping behaviors seen among trauma survivors (Machtinger et al., 2015).

Due to the stigma associated with sexual or intimate partner violence, many victims remain silent. Illness, medical procedures, treatments, and hospitalizations may be traumatic for people, and reactions from past experiences may confound current events. Medical exams can feel invasive: We ask sensitive questions, examine our patients' bodies, and sometimes perform painful procedures (Reeves & Humphreys, 2017).

Distressing healthcare experiences can act as a barrier to accessing the help the victim may need; past healthcare experiences may complicate the current experience and impact clinical practice (Reeves & Humphreys, 2017). It is imperative for the forensic nurse to recognize the risk of revictimization to the person by elements of routine care such as physical touch, supine positioning, and the power imbalance between provider and patient. The healthcare environment supports providers and contributes to the power differential between staff and patients (Machtinger et al., 2015). Trauma survivors are actively working to cope with traumatic events and make sense of them, and they are at high risk for experiencing trauma symptoms and triggers from healthcare procedures and examinations (Reeves & Humphreys, 2017).

TIC is a shift to a culture of safety, empowerment, and healing. The first step is to recognize how common trauma is, assume each patient may have a trauma history, and provide care from a trauma-informed perspective. Interventions to create safety and privacy include the following (Blanche, 2012; Reeves & Humphreys, 2017; Stokes et al., 2017):

- Give patients a choice of where in the room to sit or stand.
- Ask permission before touching or interviewing.
- Interview before they disrobe.
- Explain all medical terms and procedures.

TRAUMA ACROSS THE LIFE SPAN

Adverse childhood experiences (ACEs) are stressful or traumatic events that children experience before the age of 18, such as violence at home, neglect, abuse, or having a parent suffering from mental illness or a substance abuse habit. Frequent exposure to ACEs influences a child's response to stress, and if the exposure is severe or chronic, it can impact physical and behavioral health long into adulthood (Withers, 2017). Childhood and adult trauma have been shown to be major risk factors for the most common causes of adult illness, death, and disability in the United States (Felitti, 2009).

The 1998 Adverse Childhood Experiences Study (ACE Study) examined the relationship between chronic childhood stress and adversity and its impact on long-term health outcomes (Blanche, 2012; Felitti, 2009). In the study, researchers assigned an "ACE score" to each participant by adding up the number of adversities the participant reported. The ACE study reported two important findings:

- ACEs are incredibly common.
- The more ACEs, the higher the risk for chronic disease in adulthood.

Early traumatic experiences can alter a person's psychological and physiological development and may contribute to increased risk behaviors. Prolonged trauma may destabilize a patient's sense of safety, self, and self-efficacy and impact his or her ability to moderate emotions and navigate personal relationships (Machtinger et al., 2015).

Healthcare providers are in a unique position to screen for ACEs (see Exhibit 5.1), identify the trauma, and provide care through a "trauma-informed lens" (Withers, 2017). This requires us to listen to our patients and explore how relationships and health are affected by witnessing or experiencing abuse or other ACEs.

There is an abundance of evidence linking trauma to health outcomes (Blanche, 2012; CDC, 2014, 2017; Machtinger et al., 2015). Empowering patients to understand that childhood and adult trauma may lie beneath many illnesses and unhealthy behaviors will help our patients to move forward to physical and psychological wellness.

CAREGIVER SUPPORT AND WELL-BEING

Trauma is our life story: As the care providers who interact with patients during these life-changing events, we experience repeated or extreme exposure to graphic details and we provide care to patients during these traumatic events (Machtinger et al., 2015). A critical component of TIC is attending to the emotional needs of the caregiver. Self-care will help to prevent compassion fatigue. Caregivers need a place to continue the work of healing and to process the complex and challenging feelings and emotions that may arise when caring for patients in the wake of a traumatic or violent event (Stokes et al., 2017).

THE WAY FORWARD

Trauma is pervasive in our society. Victims of natural disasters are identified daily through media. Our veterans returning home were exposed to anticipated and actual life-threatening events every day. Trauma is present in our daily lives and work environments, as evidenced by major accidents, school shootings, and workplace and street violence. TIC presents healthcare and human service providers with a framework to administer tailored care that is transformative by approaching every patient with the assumption that, at some point in their lives, they may have experienced trauma (Blanche, 2012; Bowen & Murshid, 2016; Machtinger et al., 2015; Stokes et al., 2017). TIC is about empathy, compassion, care, and understanding as we experience and share our patients' stories. TIC is the lens through which we see our patients as "whole persons" with all their complexities, when they interact with us for help.

Exhibit 5.1

Finding Your ACE Score

While you were growing up, during your first 18 years of life:

1. Did a parent or other adult in the household often or very often swear at you, insult you, put you down, humiliate you, or act in a way that made you afraid that you might be physically hurt?
   Yes/No. If yes enter 1 _____

2. Did a parent or other adult in the household often or very often push, grab, slap, throw something at you, or ever hit you so hard that you had marks or were injured?
   Yes/No. If yes enter 1 _____

3. Did an adult or person at least 5 years older than you ever touch or fondle you; have you touch his or her body in a sexual way; or attempt or actually have oral, anal, or vaginal intercourse with you?
   Yes/No. If yes enter 1 _____

4. Did you often or very often feel that no one in your family loved you or thought you were important or special? Or did you feel your family did not look out for each other, feel close to each other, or support each other?
   Yes/No. If yes enter 1 _____

(continued)

Exhibit 5.1

Finding Your ACE Score (*continued*)

5. Did you often or very often feel that you did not have enough to eat, had to wear dirty clothes, and had no one to protect you? Or were your parents too drunk or high to take care of you or take you to the doctor if you needed it?
   Yes/No. If yes enter 1 _____

6. Were your parents ever separated or divorced?
   Yes/No. If yes enter 1 _____

7. Was your mother or stepmother often or very often pushed, grabbed, slapped, or had something thrown at her; sometimes, often, or very often kicked, bitten, hit with a fist, or hit with something hard; or ever repeatedly hit at least a few minutes or threatened with a gun or knife?
   Yes/No. If yes enter 1 _____

8. Did you live with anyone who was a problem drinker or alcoholic or who used street drugs?
   Yes/No. If yes enter 1 _____

9. Was a household member depressed or mentally ill, or did a household member attempt suicide?
   Yes/No. If yes enter 1 _____

10. Did a household member go to prison?
    Yes/No. If yes enter 1 _____
    Now add up your yes answers: _____ This is your ACE score.

ACE, adverse childhood experiences.
Source: Got your ACE score? What's your ACE score? (And, at the end, what's your resilience score?). Retrieved from https://acestoohigh.com/got-your-ace-score/

CONCLUSION

Using a trauma-informed approach to care for patients in any clinical setting is a critical aspect in nursing care. Trauma is pervasive and impacts many people from early childhood into their older years. Not all patients will disclose a trauma background yet may have lingering medical and mental health effects. Nurses are key in developing therapeutic and healing relationships with patients, which can easily start by implementing a TIC approach to all patients.

RESOURCES

Center for Youth Wellness: https://centerforyouthwellness.org/ace-toxic-stress
The Adverse Childhood Experiences Study: https://www.cdc.gov/violence prevention/acestudy/index.html
U.S. Department of Defense: Office on Violence Against Women: https://www.justice.gov/ovw
U.S. Department of Health and Human Services: Substance Abuse and Mental Health Services Administration (SAMHSA), National

Center for Trauma-Informed Care: https://www.samhsa.gov/nctic /trauma-interventions

TEDMED Talk: *How childhood trauma affects health across a lifetime* | Nadine Burke Harris: https://www.youtube.com/watch?v=95ovIJ3dsNk &feature=youtu.be

References

Blanch, A. (2012). *SAMHSA'S National Center for Trauma Informed Care: Changing communities, changing lives: Substance abuse and mental health services administration*. Rockville, MD: Substance Abuse and Mental Health Services Administration. Retrieved from https://www.nasmhpd.org/sites/default/files/NCTIC_Marketing_Brochure_FINAL(2).pdf

Bowen, E. A., & Murshid, S. M. (2016). Trauma-informed social policy: A conceptual framework for policy analysis and advocacy. *Perspectives from the Social Sciences, 106*(2), 223–229. doi:10.2105/AJPH.2015.302970

Felitti, V. J. (2009). Adverse childhood experiences and adult health. *Academic Pediatrics, 9*, 131–132. doi:10.1016/j.acap.2009.03.001

Machtinger, E. L., Cuca, Y. P., Khanna, N., Rose, C. D., & Kimberg, L. S. (2015). From treatment to healing: The promise of trauma-informed primary care. *Women's Health Issues, 25*(3), 193–197. doi:10.1016/j.whi.2015.03.008

National Center for Injury Prevention and Control, Centers for Disease Control and Prevention. (2014). Child maltreatment: Facts at a glance. Retrieved from https://www.cdc.gov/violenceprevention/pdf/childmaltreatment-facts-at-a-glance.pdf

National Center for Injury Prevention and Control, Centers for Disease Control and Prevention. (2017). Findings from the National Intimate Partner and Sexual Violence Survey. Retrieved from https://www.cdc.gov/violenceprevention/pdf/NISVS-StateReportFactsheet.pdf

Reeves, E. A., & Humphreys, J. C. (2017). Describing the healthcare experiences and strategies of women survivors of violence. *Journal of Clinical Nursing, 27*, 1170–1182. doi:10.1111/jocn.14152

Stokes, Y., Jacob, J. D., Gifford, W., Squires, J., & Vandyk, A. (2017). Exploring nurses' knowledge and experiences related to trauma-informed care. *Global Qualitative Nursing Research, 4*, 1–10. doi:10.1177/2333393617734510

Wilson, C. (2013). More psychologists with training in trauma needed: Psychologists gather experts to develop a core competency model in trauma care. *Monitor on Psychology, 44*(8), 36. Retrieved from http://www.apa.org/monitor/2013/09/index.aspx

II

Issues of Sexual and Interpersonal Violence

6

Sexual Assault

Meredith J. Scannell

Sexual assault is a major public health problem that occurs across all demographic, socioeconomic, and racial groups. Understanding the complexity of sexual violence and the unique healthcare needs of victims of sexual violence is essential for forensic nurses and many healthcare providers. Patients who have been sexually assaulted may have direct medical, psychological, legal, and forensic needs. Having an understanding of the different aspects of caring for victims of sexual assault will allow for healthcare providers to provide care that will improve health outcome and decrease further victimization.

At the end of the chapter, the nurse will be able to:

1. Understand the epidemiological aspect of sexual assault.
2. Understand the unique healthcare needs of patients who have been sexually assaulted.
3. Describe the different prophylactic medications for sexually transmitted infections (STIs) and pregnancy.
4. Recognize the need for prompt HIV postexposure prophylaxis.
5. Explain the need for follow-up care.

BACKGROUND

The National Crime Victimization Survey (NCVS) is one of the most reliable surveys that determines the rates of sexual assault in the United States. According to the latest report, 431,840 individuals were sexually assaulted in 2015 (Truman & Morgan, 2016). These numbers are often an underestimation, as not all victims will disclose a sexual assault. Of the reported sexual assaults, 28% were noted to be complete rapes, 21% attempted rapes, 27% sexual assaults, 6% unwanted contact without force, and 17% were verbal threats of rape and sexual assault (Truman & Morgan, 2016).

Sexual assault is defined by the U.S. Department of Justice as any type of sexual contact or behavior that occurs without the explicit consent of the recipient, including acts such as forced sexual intercourse, forcible sodomy, child molestation, incest, fondling, pornography, and attempted rape. Rape has a narrow definition and relates to nonconsensual penetration of the vagina, anus, or mouth with the use of force, coercion, or threats of bodily harm, including victims who are incapacitated or unable to give consent.

The Centers for Disease Control (CDC) and Prevention has defined the different types of sexual violence listed in Table 6.1.

Table 6.1

Sexual Assault Definitions

Types of Sexual Assaults	Definition
Penetration assault (rape)	"Includes unwanted vaginal, oral, or anal insertion through use of physical force or threats to bring physical harm toward or against the victim."
Drug-facilitated assault	"Includes unwanted vaginal, oral, or anal insertion when the victim was unable to consent because he or she was too intoxicated (e.g., unconscious, or lack of awareness) through voluntary or involuntary use of alcohol or drugs."
Unwanted sexual contact	"Includes intentional touching, either directly or through the clothing, of the genitalia, anus, groin, breast, inner thigh, or buttocks of any person without his or her consent, or of a person who is unable to consent. Unwanted sexual contact also includes making a victim touch the perpetrator."
Noncontact unwanted sexual experiences	"Includes unwanted sexual attention that does not involve physical contact. Some examples are verbal sexual harassment (e.g., making sexual comments) or unwanted exposure to pornography. This occurs without a person's consent and sometimes, without the victim's knowledge."

Source: Centers for Disease Control and Prevention. (2018, April 10). Sexual violence: Definitions. Retrieved from https://www.cdc.gov/violenceprevention/sexualviolence/definitions.html

Fast Facts

Penetration includes any type of insertion, even "minimal" or "slight." It does not have to be a complete insertion.

Victims who have been sexually assaulted have historically faced a negative reaction from police, law enforcement, healthcare agencies, counselors, and even their own friends, families, and colleagues. It is often termed "victim blaming" and stems from rape myths: beliefs that are imbedded throughout society that victims are responsible for the assault and that acts against them are justified. These negative reactions result in secondary victimization whereby the individual who has been sexually assaulted becomes a victim again from the negative response around them. When this occurs, victims are more likely to develop negative reactions such as guilt, self-blame, and depression, are less likely to trust others and their services, and are less likely to seek further help. They are also less likely to engage in legal proceedings.

Different communities may experience different degrees of victim blaming. For example, stigma and homophobic discriminatory behaviors can be a barrier for individuals within the lesbian, gay, bisexual, and transsexual communities to report and seek help for services after a sexual assault. Men feel that they will not be believed or that they asked for the assault because of misconceptions that men who have sex with men are promiscuous or that sexual assaults cannot happen to men.

In an effort to address and improve responses to victims of sexual assault, specialized interdisciplinary teams and nurses have been developed, such as sexual assault response teams (SARTs) and sexual assault nurse examiners (SANEs; Lynch, 2011). SARTs are multi-disciplinary teams of professionals who work together in responding to victims' legal, medical, and social needs. Members of SART can include law enforcement officials, sexual assault detectives, prosecutors, healthcare professionals, forensic nurses, counselors, and social workers (Lynch, 2011). They work together in providing care to victims of sexual assault so that the response is coordinated and seamless. There are different SART models of care, including community-based or hospital-based teams. The goal is to prioritize victims' care and hold perpetrators accountable for the assault. SANEs are registered nurses who may work with SARTs, individually or within healthcare systems. They have undergone specialized education and training and can provide nursing care and assessments along with performing medical forensic evaluation and evidence collection for victims of sexual assault. Although there remain gaps in services for sexually assaulted patients, the development and implementation of specialized services have resulted in improvements to the responses for sexual assault victims.

HEALTHCARE NEEDS

Victims of sexual assault have unique healthcare needs and require an individualized approach to treating time (Lynch, 2011). Treatment is often guided by the acts that occurred, when they occurred, the severity of injuries, the healthcare provider's recommendations, and the patient's preference for treatment. The first aspect of care for victims is a medical assessment and physical exam, especially for any life-threatening injuries. During the assault, serious injuries could have been inflicted and a focused medical assessment should address life-threatening, serious, or time-sensitive injuries first. Depending on the severity of the injury, it may be best to wait to treat the injury until evidence collection is completed. All injuries warrant careful documentation and some may be in different stages of healing (Henry, 2012).

Some common injuries sustained in sexual assaults include bite marks, which can result in an imprint of the assailant's teeth or a mark from suction that was applied with the bite (Henry, 2012). Defensive wounds often appear on the backs of arms when they are being held up in an attempt to shield from violence (Henry, 2012). Pattern injuries can also appear, which result in an injury that takes on the appearance of the weapon used, such as fingerprints, or patterns of the sole of the assailant's shoe. Victims who have been strangled may have fingerprints on their necks or a ligature mark that encircles the entire neck depending on the mechanism of violence. Common areas for anovaginal injuries include the fossa navicularis, posterior fourchette, labia minora, perineum, vagina, cervix, and anus (Jones, Rossman, Hartman, & Alexander, 2003). All injuries should be carefully documented, in case of legal prosecution or for continuous evaluation of injuries that take a long time to heal such that progress can be monitored. A body diagram map should be used for documenting injuries to demonstrate where they occurred on the body.

SEXUALLY TRANSMITTED INFECTIONS

Being exposed to STIs is a serious sequela of sexual assault and victims may require prophylactic treatment depending on the acts committed. Patients who have sustained assault where they have been exposed to STIs should be given all recommended prophylactic medications (CDC, 2016). Testing practices for STIs among sexually assaulted patients vary across healthcare organizations, where some practices are to test for STIs among all victims and other practices will treat prophylaticaly for STI's without testing. Practices for HIV testing will vary by institution and sexual assault protocols, as some healthcare institutions will recommend baseline testing and others will recommend HIV testing after 6 weeks to determine seroconversion. Patients with unknown hepatitis B status or unsure status will need to have titers drawn to determine the correct postexposure regimen.

All patients with possible exposure to STIs should receive prophylactic treatment for gonorrhea, chlamydia, and trichomonas, the most common bacterial infections, and treatment for these STIs is a one-time dose given in the acute setting. Possible exposure to HIV is a significant concern for many patients. Unlike the other prophylactic medications, HIV prophylaxis is time sensitive and a 28-day course of antivirals should be given as soon as possible (Scannell, Kim, & Guthrie, 2018). Patients receiving HIV prophylaxis will require a baseline liver function test and blood counts for the duration of the HIV prophylactic therapy to monitor for adverse medication effects. A recent update to the 2016 CDC guidelines issued a caution in using the antiretroviral dolutegravir in pregnancy, as it has recently been shown to have a teratogenic effect on the newborn.

Hepatitis B vaccination status should be verified for all patients who present for care (Table 6.2). A complete postexposure hepatitis B vaccine series should be given in the acute period for patients with no hepatitis B immunity. Human papillomavirus (HPV) is one of the most common STIs and current updates recommend that sexually assaulted patients receive the HPV vaccine if not contraindicated.

Fast Facts

A sexually assaulted patient receives a lot of medicine and may need an antiemetic prior to taking all medications.

TETANUS

The patient's tetanus status should also be assessed. If the patient has not had a tetanus toxoid vaccine within the last 5 years, he or she should receive the tetanus toxoid booster. The risk of tetanus increases if there are open cuts or even microabrasions present. Assess the victim for injuries that may have occurred outside, or dirty/rust objects that were used during the assault that places the

Table 6.2

Prophylactic Treatment Recommendations

Infection/Condition	Recommended Treatment Within 5 Days	5 Days–2 Weeks Postassault	1–2 Months Postassault	2–6 Months Postassault
Neisseria gonorrhoeae	Provide prophylactic treatment if it was not given Ceftriaxone 250 mg IM single dose	Test for STIs, treat if positive		
Chlamydia trachomatis	Provide prophylactic treatment if it was not given Azithromycin 1 gm PO single dose	Test for STIs, treat if positive		
Trichomoniasis	Metronidazole (2 g orally in a single dose)	Test for trichomoniasis and provide prophylactic treatment if positive test results		
Unvaccinated individual and hepatitis B positive assailant	Administer first dose of hepatitis B vaccine series and HBSIG		Administer the second dose at 1–2 months	Administer the third dose at 4–6 months
Unvaccinated individual and assailant hepatitis B status unknown	Administer first dose of hepatitis B vaccine		Administer the second dose at 1–2 months	Administer the third dose at 4–6 months
Previously vaccinated	Consider giving hepatitis B booster if needed			
(HIV)				
≥18 years of age with a negative urine pregnancy test, normal liver function, complete blood count tests, and a creatinine clearance of ≥50 mL/min	Emtricitabine/tenofovir—one tablet orally every day for 28 days—plus lopinavir/ritonivir—two tablets orally twice daily for 28 days. Patients with baseline abnormal renal function should not receive emtricitabine/tenofovir, give lopinavir/ritonavir plus lamivudine/zidovudine with dosing adjustments	Offer counseling if no prophylaxis was given and ask to return in 6 weeks postassault for HIV testing	HIV testing at 6 weeks postassault	HIV testing at 6 months

≥12 years of age and <18 years of age or is pregnant at any age with normal liver function and complete blood count tests and a creatinine clearance of ≥50 mL/min	Lamivudine/zidovudine—one tablet orally twice daily for 28 days—and lopinavir/ritonavir—two tablets by mouth twice daily for 28 days		
Tetanus	Tetanus booster (if indicated)	Tetanus booster (if indicated) and not given previously	
Pregnancy	Levonorgestrel (Plan B) 1.5 mg orally in a single dose or 0.75 mg orally in split dose 12 hr apart or ulipristal acetate 30 mg in a single dose Consider copper IUD for individuals with high BMI	Perform pregnancy testing if no pregnancy prophylaxis was given within 5 days of the assault	Perform pregnancy testing if received prophylaxis and have not had menstrual cycle
HPV	Recommended for females aged 9–26: administer first dose of HPV vaccine series	Administer second dose at 1–2 months after the first dose	Administer third dose at 6 months. If first dose was not given, discuss options for HPV vaccine with patient

BMI, body mass index; HBSIG, hepatitis B-specific immunoglobulin; HPV, human papillomavirus; IM, intramuscular; IUD, intrauterine device; PO, per os; STI, sexually transmitted infection.

Source: American College of Emergency Physicians. (2013). *Evaluation and management of the sexually assaulted or sexually abused patient*. Dallas, TX: American College of Emergency Physicians; Centers for Disease Control and Prevention. (2016). Updated guidelines for antiretroviral post exposure prophylaxis after sexual, injection drug use, or other nonoccupational exposure to HIV—United States, 2016. *Annals of Emergency Medicine*, 68(3), 335–338. doi:10.1016/j.annemergmed.2016.06.028

victim at risk for the transmission of tetanus. There is no contraindication to receiving multiple vaccines, though the sites of administration should differ.

PREGNANCY TESTING AND PROPHYLAXIS

All patients who present for care within 5 days of an assault should have a pregnancy test. A positive pregnancy test may impact the treatment, medications prescribed, and course of care. Pregnancy prophylaxis (emergency contraception) is a standard of care for women who have been sexually assaulted and should be offered to all women where it is not contraindicated. Emergency contraception comes in two forms: oral hormonal methods, such as levonorgestrel and ulipristal acetate, and copper intrauterine devices (IUDs). Hormones are administered as either a single- or two-dose treatment. The single dose is the preferred method and can be taken up to 120 hours after the assault (Praditpan, et al., 2017). Levonorgestrel, a progestin, is best given within 2 days due to a decrease in efficacy with time (Praditpan, et al., 2017). The antiprogestin ulipristal acetate can be given up to 120 hours after exposure and maintains its efficacy in preventing a pregnancy (Praditpan, et al., 2017). Another option for emergency contraception is the copper IUD, which is the most effective method of emergency contraception and can be inserted up to 5 days after exposure. Contraindication for the IUD is females with extensive vaginal and cervical injuries that may have occurred during the assault. For females who present after 120 hours, they should be counseled about the risk of pregnancy and offered pregnancy testing at that time and 1 month later if no menstrual cycle has occurred.

MENTAL HEALTHCARE

Sexual assault can cause acute and long-term psychological trauma (Lynch, 2011). All victims should be assessed for adverse psychological outcomes during the acute phase and throughout the treatment and recovery period. Adverse psychological outcomes include:

- Posttraumatic stress disorder (PTSD)
- Depression
- Anxiety
- Suicidal ideation
- Excessive or problematic drinking
- Substance use
- Nonmedical use of prescription drugs
- Engagement in risky health behaviors
- Rape trauma syndrome

When compared to other traumatic events, women who have sustained a sexual assault have significantly more PTSD symptomology. This is concerning because researchers have noted a possible mediating relationship between PTSD and risky health behaviors as well as risk for subsequent sexual assault. Often these adverse psychological outcomes are multifaceted and occur in conjunction with each other.

FOLLOW-UP CARE

Follow-up care is an essential aspect of healthcare for patients who have been sexually assaulted and should be ongoing throughout the recovery period. Patients may need additional treatment for injuries, medications or vaccines, testing for STIs and pregnancy, evaluation of side effects of medications or the efficacy of medications, and reassessment for possible diseases and mental health assessments. All patients should be informed of immediate signs and symptoms that require medical attention and signs and symptoms of specific STIs, as some antibiotics and antivirals may not prevent the disease. If possible, a follow-up appointment should be made during the first visit to encourage the patient to return for further care. Written information should include details of the services provided, including what medications or prescriptions the patient received. Patients should be instructed on signs and symptoms of STIs and written instructions should be given for reinforcement. Support and information on advocacy services should also be provided.

HIV nonoccupational postexposure (n-PEP) starter packs typically consisting of 3 to 5 days of antiviral medications are given to patients who present in an emergency room. Starter packs may be phased out, as CDC guidelines recommend a 28-day prescription given the higher completion rates (CDC, 2016).

Fast Facts

HIV n-PEP compliance is often poor among sexually assaulted patients and counseling regarding adherence is essential.

Follow-up care is essential for patients who have been prescribed this medication, to monitor abnormal laboratory levels and to prescribe the remainder of the medications. Patients who receive these medications should be counseled on their risk of acquiring HIV and the importance of adherence (Scannell, Kim, & Guthrie, 2018). Reasons for nonadherence should be addressed. All patients who present outside the 72-hour window for n-PEP should be counseled on their risk of HIV and tested. Whether patients receive n-PEP or not, they should be counseled and tested for HIV at 6 weeks and 6 months.

COUNSELING

Many patients will benefit from rape counseling and advocacy in the aftermath of a sexual assault. Several local and national programs have been developed to help meet the needs of victims of violence. Different organizations have been developed to meet specific patient populations that understand and address their unique healthcare and mental health needs.

RAPE, ABUSE, AND INCEST NATIONAL NETWORK

The Rape, Abuse, and Incest National Network (RAINN) is the largest organization in the United States that has partnerships with other national and local organizations to provide services to victims of sexual assault. They have a free telephone hotline [1-800-656-HOPE(4673)] and web hotline that victims can call and have access to free help. The organization also has resources and information for different communities disproportionately affected by sexual violence and additional resources and training materials for healthcare providers who work with victims of sexual assault.

FOLLOW-UP INSTRUCTIONS

- Provide patients with discharge instructions indicating which medication they received for care.
- Schedule a follow-up appointment with the healthcare provider or HIV specialist if additional medications need to be prescribed.
- Encourage the patient to seek mental health services postassault with either a new provider or an established one to help with the recovery process.
- If emergency contraception was declined, instruct the patient to have a repeat pregnancy test in 10 to 14 days and repeat in 1 month, especially if menses has not occurred.
- Instruct the patient on the importance of HIV postexposure adherence, as nonadherence can result in medication failure.

REPORTING TO LAW ENFORCEMENT

Reporting a sexual assault to law enforcement is up to the victim. Although reporting to the police may make the case stronger, there are valid reasons why a victim may not report the case to the police. One genuine fear is retaliation from the perpetrator, and that the perpetrator will find out that a report was made and will then retaliate against the patient. Other common reasons victims do not report can be that they are often embarrassed, worried about privacy, or fearful of punishment for other illegal issues such as underage drinking or illicit substance use (Lonsway, Archambault, & Berger, 2000). Other reasons can be a fear of the police and that reporting will cause a secondary victimization in which they then are traumatized further.

SAFETY

Safety is always a priority for patients who have been sexually assaulted (Lonsway, Archambault, & Berger, 2000). Safety planning may be a necessary component of patient care as many sexual assaults are committed by someone who is known to the victim and the fear of retaliation can be a genuine concern. Ensuring safety may mean contacting local police enforcement (if the patient agrees) and filing a restraining order. In some cases where sexual violence occurs with an intimate partner, the individual may need help with accessing a shelter or making an escape plan (Lonsway, Archambault, & Berger, 2000).

CONCLUSION

Sexual assault remains a serious public health problem that impacts the lives of both female and male adults and children. Although evidence supports the use of SANE and SART programs, they are not always available. Healthcare professionals must be trained and educated about the complexities and needs of sexually assaulted patients so that the healthcare community can take an active role in helping to identify those at risk so they can treat and address the issue.

References

American College of Emergency Physicians. (2013). *Evaluation and management of the sexually assaulted or sexually abused patient.* Dallas, TX: American College of Emergency Physicians.

Centers for Disease Control and Prevention. (2016). Updated guidelines for antiretroviral post exposure prophylaxis after sexual, injection drug use, or other nonoccupational exposure to HIV—United States, 2016. *Annals of Emergency Medicine, 68*(3), 335–338. doi:10.1016/j. annemergmed.2016.06.028

Centers for Disease Control and Prevention. (2018, April 10). Sexual violence: Definitions. Retrieved from https://www.cdc.gov/violenceprevention/sexualviolence/definitions.html

Henry, T. (2012). *Atlas of sexual violence*. St. Louis, MO: Elsevier Mosby.

Jones, J. S., Rossman, L., Hartman, M., & Alexander, C. C. (2003). Anogenital injuries in adolescents after consensual sexual intercourse. *Academic Emergency Medicine*, *10*(12), 1378–1383. doi:10.1197/S1069-6563(03)00555-4

Lonsway, K., Archambault, J., & Berger, R. (2000). Successfully investigating acquaintance sexual assault: A national training manual for law enforcement. *National Center for Women & Policing, Office of Justice Programs (Grant# 97-WE-VX-K004)*.

Lynch, V., & Duval, J. B. (2011). *Forensic nursing science* (2nd ed.). St. Louis, MO: Mosby/Elsevier.

Praditpan, P., Hamouie, A., Basaraba, C. N., Nandakumar, R., Cremers, S., Davis, A. R., & Westhoff, C. L. (2017). Pharmacokinetics of levonorgestrel and ulipristal acetate emergency contraception in women with normal and obese body mass index. *Contraception*, *95*(5), 464–469. doi:10.1016/j.contraception.2017.01.004

Scannell, M., Kim, T., & Guthrie, B. J. (2018). A meta-analysis of HIV postexposure prophylaxis among sexually assaulted patients in the United States. *Journal of the Association of Nurses in AIDS Care*, *29*(1), 60–69. doi:10.1016/j.jana.2017.10.004

Truman, J. L., & Morgan, R. E. (2016). *Criminal victimization, 2015*. Retrieved from https://www.bjs.gov/content/pub/pdf/cv15.pdf

U.S. Department of Justice, Office on Violence Against Women. (2013). *National protocol for sexual assault medical forensic examinations: Adults/adolescents* (2nd ed.). Washington, DC: Author.

7

Military Sexual Trauma

Meredith J. Scannell

Sexual violence occurs in a variety of settings, including in the military. Unlike other settings, the military culture can impact victims of sexual violence. Forensic nurses can play a key role in addressing issues of military sexual violence in a manner that is confidential and supportive to patients. In addition, forensic nurses are able to pick up on red flags and signs of sexual violence and harassment that may go unnoticed and help to address an underserved group of patients at high risk for suicide.

At the end of the chapter, the nurse will be able to:

1. Understand the scope of military sexual trauma (MST).
2. Describe how the culture of the military impacts victims of sexual violence and harassment.
3. Describe how MST relates to increased risk of suicide.

BACKGROUND

MST is a term used to cover different forms of sexual violence, including sexual harassment and sexual assault that has occurred during active duty, active duty training, or inactive duty training (Castro, Kintzle, Schuyler, Lucas, & Warner, 2015). MST is recognized as a hazard of being employed in the U.S. military services. A large meta-analysis by Wilson (2016) found 15.7% of military personnel and veterans reporting MST of both sexual harassment and sexual assault, with women disproportionately affected (38.4%) compared to men (3.9%).

EXAMPLES OF MST

- Offensive remarks about a person's body or sexual activities
- Threatening and unwelcome sexual advances
- Unwanted touching or grabbing
- Oral sex, anal sex, sexual penetration with an object and/or sexual intercourse without the person's consent
- Taking pictures or videos of an individual without his or her consent
- Forcing or pressuring something sexual for workplace benefit
- Asking about the individual's sexual activities
- Repeatedly being told of not acting according to one's gender role

MST occurs in all branches of the military. In 2014 the RAND National Defense Research Institute workplace report found rates of sexual assault across all ranks of military personnel with higher rates of MST have been reported; more often the assailant is a service member of higher rank or supervisor of the unit. Most often MST occurs on a military installation or ship, followed by at sea or during field exercises, in a civilian location, deployment in a compact location, and least at basic training. This same report found that of active women in the service, those in the marine corps have the highest percentage experiencing sexual assault (19.48%), followed by the navy (16.71%), the army (14.49%), and lastly the air force (11.94%). The percentage of active males in the service was highest among the navy (3.37%), followed by the marine corps (2.12%), the army (1.95%), and least among the air force (1.05%).

HEALTH IMPLICATIONS

Military service personnel experience many traumatic stressors, especially when deployed. Unlike other military traumatic stressors, MST is often perpetrated by someone within the military services (Castro, Kintzle, Schuyler, Lucas, & Warner, 2015). Individuals are then faced with several traumas: being in the military; job-related stressors; and then the added stress of MST. Service men and women who have experienced MST go on to have significant mental health sequelae including depression, posttraumatic stress disorders, substance misuse and abuse, and suicide ideation. Suicide ideation is a significant finding among service men and women with histories of MST, when compared to those without MST histories, and they are more likely to have made a suicide attempt.

Fast Facts

MST has been directly related to significant mental health disorders, including the development of PTSD and numerous mental health concerns such as anxiety, depression, and suicide ideation and suicide attempts.

When individuals experience trauma, the body responds and adapts to the trauma and activates the fight, flight, or freeze stress response. This stress response is a physiological activation that is hormonal, neurological, physiological, and emotional and allows the individual to deal with the acute traumatic stress. Over time the physiological impact of trauma has a direct impact on the neurobiology of the individual, affecting his or her mental health, such as impaired memory recall and hyperarousal. For military service personnel who work in high-security or combat areas, this can have a negative impact on their ability to function optimally in their responsibilities. MST can impact the day-to-day activities of service members, which then impact their ability to adhere to military duties.

MILITARY CULTURAL ISSUES RELATED TO MST

- Team allegiance, looked down upon to report anything negative about the team or unit, including reporting MST
- Changing units, assignments, or locations, which creates an opportunist environment, victimizes an individual right before or right after their changed unit, assignment, or location
- Living arrangements in co-ed dorms and rooms make the area high risk
- The same institution is responsible for the care of the victim and assailant
- High value placed on strength and self-sufficiency
- Addressing MST may disrupt career goals
- MST is a women's issue

Addressing MST is now a priority of the U.S. government, which, with the Veterans Administration, implements mandatory screening for active duty military and veterans, in addition to increasing treatment services. In 2005 a congressional mandate enacted the Department of Defense Sexual Assault Prevention and Responsibility Policy. Part of the mandate is to track the number of sexual assault and sexual harassment cases that occur and are prosecuted each year.

The Sexual Assault Prevention and Response Office (SAPRO) is the authoritative division that oversees the implementation and regulation of the sexual assault policy. The SAPRO provides resources, training kits, and reporting guidelines.

CLINICAL IMPLICATIONS

Service men and women may present for care at military and non-military healthcare centers, seeking care post MST. Circumstances specific to being in the military may make it difficult for someone to report an MST, as it may result in additional stress and stigma and may mean the end of one's career or promotion. As forensic nurses we must consider the unique circumstances of military personnel when providing care. When caring for victims who have experienced MST, it is essential to screen for suicide ideation, especially among males, who have a significantly higher rate of suicide attempts with histories of MST.

In addition, having experienced trauma will directly impact how one will seek out healthcare, and this places emphasis on the need to screen everyone for MST; however, they present themselves seeking healthcare. Many victims will not disclose MST unless directly asked. Universal screening will help identify individuals who have experienced MST and are seeking healthcare for a different health condition. Universal screening is especially helpful and has identified cases of MST among service individuals who were seeking mental healthcare services for the first time. This illustrates the importance of universal screening and should be part of care, especially for those who may have other red flags, such as suicide ideation or medical conditions such as sexually transmitted infections (STIs) or unwanted pregnancies.

REPORTING MST

Two options are available for MST reporting: restricted and unrestricted. Restricted reporting is an option for active duty military personnel and certain criteria must be met. Unrestricted reporting initiates the criminal process. Reporting MST is often complex and difficult for service men and women. Many of the perpetrators are in the military services as well and there may be many factors that make it difficult to report MST. Power dynamics may play a pivotal role in keeping a victim from reporting MST as many victims are subordinates, dependent upon, or may directly report to their perpetrators. This power dynamic makes it difficult to report for fear

BOX 7.1 MILITARY CULTURAL ISSUES THAT IMPACT MST

- Stigma-related barriers
- Not wanting to talk about problems
- Embarrassment or shame
- Privacy/confidentiality
- Self-blame
- Not important or serious enough
- Sensitivity and reactions of a provider
- Fear that they will not be believed
- Gender-related barriers
- Rape myth belief that men are less affected than women
- Masculinity or male pride would be diminished if reported or sought help
- Sexuality and sexual orientation and concerns how others will perceive them
- Provider gender preferences
- Knowledge barriers
- Lack of knowledge about service availability
- Financial concerns regarding services

Source: Turchik, J. A., McLean, C., Rafie, S., Hoyt, T., Rosen, C. S., & Kimerling, R. (2013). Perceived barriers to care and provider gender preferences among veteran men who have experienced military sexual trauma: A qualitative analysis. *Psychological Services, 10*(2), 213. doi:10.1037/a0029959; Morral, A. R., Gore, K. L., & Schell, T. L. (2015). *Sexual assault and sexual harassment in the US Military. Volume 2. Estimates for department of defense service members from the 2014 RAND Military Workplace Study*. Santa Monica, CA: Rand National Defense Research Inst.

of retaliation. The assault may occur overseas with an assailant who is a service person of the same rank and someone who needs to be depended on during combat. Even when the individual does bring MST to the attention of someone, he or she often experiences a negative outcome—being told to drop the issue, being retaliated against, being discouraged from filing a formal complaint, and even being assigned to a less favorable job or denied promotion.

REASONS MST NOT REPORTED

- Lack of confidentiality, especially among small groups where it is easily identified that the individual reporting the incident would be the only female in the group

- Lack of sexual assault reporting services, especially when deployed
- Pressure to maintain group cohesiveness, and reporting will break up the group
- Negative reactions and perceptions from friends, peers, and family
- Self-blame or fear of retaliation
- Military career may be affected
- Encouraged to remain silent
- Worried about retaliation
- The act would be minimized
- Want to forget about the incident and move on

FOLLOW-UP CARE

Anyone who reports MST or is having care after a MST should have ongoing follow-up care. Part of the follow-up care should include mental health resources, support systems, and safety plans that are aimed at reducing the risk for suicide ideation. One of the barriers noted in military individuals seeking care was a lack of knowledge. Having outreach programs that inform others of available services and what the services are and where they are located would help reach many individuals who have little knowledge of MST services.

CONCLUSION

MST is a serious problem that affects the lives of those who have committed to serving others. Having the skills to identify, treat, and refer may be instrumental in the health outcomes of military individuals who often will have increased risk of suicide. Further research into best follow-up care practices and outreach programs in reducing negative health outcomes may be critical in gaining necessary support. Forensic nurses can be champions in addressing this need and advocating for a vulnerable group of people.

RESOURCES

Military Rape Crisis Center: http://militaryrapecrisiscenter.org
My Duty to Speak: http://mydutytospeak
National Center on Domestic and Sexual Violence: http://www.ncdsv.org
National Center for PTSD at the U.S. Department of Veteran Affairs: http://www.ptsd.va.gov
National Sexual Violence Resource Center: http://www.nsvrc.org
Sexual Assault Prevention and Response Office (SAPRO): http://sapr.mil
Sexual Harassment/Assault Response and Prevention (SHARP) Program: http://www.sexualassault.army.mil

References

Castro, C. A., Kintzle, S., Schuyler, A. C., Lucas, C. L., & Warner, C. H. (2015). Sexual assault in the military. *Current Psychiatry Reports, 17*(7), 54. doi:10.1007/s11920-015-0596-7

Kimerling, R., Street, A. E., Gima, K., & Smith, M. W. (2008). Evaluation of universal screening for military-related sexual trauma. *Psychiatric Services, 59*(6), 635–640. doi:10.1176/ps.2008.59.6.635

Wilson, L. C. (2016). The prevalence of military sexual trauma: A meta-analysis. *Trauma, Violence, & Abuse.* Epub ahead of print. doi:10.1177/1524838016683459

8

Campus Sexual Assault

Meredith J. Scannell

Sexual assaults that occur on college campuses are a significant public health problem that impact the health and academics of the victims. The culture of colleges including fraternities, sororities, and athletics significantly impact vulnerability to sexual assault as well as perpetrators of sexual assault. In addition, the use of alcohol and rise of ride shares can impact victimization. Forensic nurses and nurses who work with college-aged students are instrumental in identifying, treating, and following up with victims and can be instrumental in educational outreach to address campus sexual assault.

At the end of the chapter, the nurse will be able to:

1. Recognize how the culture on college campuses makes students vulnerable to sexual assault.
2. Identify signs and symptoms in college students that are warning signs of a sexual assault.
3. Describe different examples of rape myths.
4. Describe how federal law is addressing campus sexual assault.

BACKGROUND

Sexual assault on college campuses and among college and university students is a significant problem. Studies have demonstrated that the rates of sexual assault among college students are as high as 28.5% (Cantor, et al., 2015). College students are significantly more likely to be victims of sexual assault compared to noncollege students, with the highest rates within the first and second semesters of school (Sinozich & Langton, 2014; Krebs, et al., 2016). Females are at a greater risk, with one in five female college students experiencing sexual assault.

A sexual assault can have medical and psychological effects, which can impact academic performance. Victims of sexual assault can sustain injuries, sexually transmitted infections, unwanted pregnancies, depression, anxiety, suicide ideation, and posttraumatic stress disorders. These negative health outcomes can have an impact on academic performance. Table 8.1 lists the medical, psychological, and academic warning signs of campus sexual assault.

Fast Facts

Approximately one in three college students who was a victim of sexual assault had academic problems and more than one in five considered leaving school altogether.

Students may need to take time away from attending classes and studying to be treated for medical conditions. The psychological

Table 8.1

Signs of Sexual Assault

Type of Sign	Warning Signs
Medical	■ Sexually transmitted infections ■ Unwanted pregnancies ■ Unexplained or poorly explained injuries ■ Defensive injuries
Psychological	■ Depression ■ Suicide ideation ■ Self-harming behaviors, such as cutting ■ Increase in substance use, especially alcohol ■ Anxiety
Academic	■ Sudden change in academic performance (lower test grades) ■ Decrease in class participation ■ Change in seats or classes (in an effort to avoid someone) ■ Missing classes ■ Withdrawing from classes or the school ■ Sudden change in school friends or social activities

impact may make studying difficult or students may want to avoid certain areas on campus or classes, especially if the perpetrator is a student and on campus.

CAMPUS CULTURE AND SEXUAL ASSAULT

The culture within the college campus places students at risk for sexual assault. One risk associated with sexual assault is alcohol consumption, which is heavily embedded in the college years and leaves students, especially females, vulnerable to sexual assault. Research conducted among college females has shown an association between high levels of alcohol consumption and sexual assault. Alcohol impacts both the perpetrator and the victim of the assault. Among perpetrators, alcohol increases aggressive behaviors and diminishes the ability to interpret cues or signs to stop (Lorenz & Ullman, 2016).

Another cultural aspect among several colleges is the "hook-up" culture, which is the socialization of casual sex among college students. Students engage in casual sex with each other to leverage their social status. Students who do not engage in the hook-up culture are then considered to have a lower social status or to be on the margins of the social scene. Hook-ups can occur in a variety of settings, such as fraternities, parties, and clubs, and often involve alcohol consumption. This behavior can send mixed messages and negative behaviors can result, such as being forced or pressured to engage in sexual activity that the individual did not want (Lorenz & Ullman, 2016). This then contributes to a rape culture whereby assaults are accepted as the social norm.

COLLEGE FRATERNITIES AND SORORITIES

College fraternities and sororities have a long history within colleges. They are organized groups formed among students who share a common goal or interest. Each group within a specific college has a subgroup known as a "chapter" with national and some international affiliation. Long-term bonds are formed among members through common experiences and group activities. Membership is often lifelong, which starts with a recruitment and initiation phase, otherwise known as the "rush" phase, and successful pledging. During the college years, the fraternity and sorority may engage in positive academic and social activities. Unfortunately, they also engage in risky behaviors and activities that can have a negative impact on health and academics. One serious negative aspect of being a member of a fraternity or sorority is the risk of sexual assault. There is a growing body of research showing a strong link between sexual assault and being a sorority member. As a sorority member, there are more social events in which alcohol is consumed and an individual is less likely to pick up on dangerous cues or may be unable to ward off or escape a predator. In addition, the sorority can have rules that restrict one's behavior, and even if a sorority member has a boyfriend, this boyfriend may not be allowed to sleep over in the sorority house. This then limits the individual and she may then have to go to the boyfriend's place of residence or fraternity, which could be an unsafe environment, especially if there are large groups of males drinking.

Examples of rape myths are as follows:

- "No" really means "yes."
- It was her fault; she was asking for it.
- It happens all the time.
- Most rapes are by strangers.
- You can tell who "wants it" by the way they act and dress.
- It's no big deal; it's just sex.
- Men cannot be sexually assaulted.
- She should have tried harder to get away.
- He just misunderstood the signals due to his drinking.
- He had sex with her before, so it is okay to do it again.
- She was giving signals that it was okay.

COLLEGE ATHLETES

Research has shown an association between sexual assaults in college students and male college athletes, especially those who play on team sports. Alcohol misuse is widely seen in male college athletes. They also have higher false rape myth beliefs about sexual assaults, victims, and perpetrators. The majority of male college athletes have high levels of self-confidence and hypermasculinity and are often considered to have a higher status, which creates a form of entitlement. Hypermasculinity is often marked by a tendency for the male to dominate and subordinate females, often through aggression, strength, drive, and ambition. These aspects then create a culture among athletes that they can do no wrong and it becomes difficult for other students to stand up against them or speak out against them when they witness sexual harassment or sexual violence, thereby reinforcing the culture of misconduct. There are also reports of college officials covering up instances of sexual violence.

RIDE SHARE SERVICES

Ride-sharing services have been a popular mechanism of transportation among college students, as they are often cheaper than regular taxi services, allow convenient pick-up and drop-up locations, and are often advertised and promoted as a safer option of transportation when drinking alcohol (Nudd, 2017; Roderick, 2016; Uber, 2017). However, less recognized is the risk factor of sexual assault, especially when a female has been drinking and gets into a ride-sharing service alone with a strange driver. It is unknown what extent of ride shares is associated with assault, as this data is not typically collected. However, there have been several cases of sexual assault occurring on college campuses in which the perpetrators are specifically looking for intoxicated students to lure them into their cars and sexually assault them (Feit, 2017; Glaser, 2018).

ADDRESSING CAMPUS SEXUAL ASSAULT

There have been several advances in addressing the problem of sexual assaults on college campus. The U.S. White House Task Force to Protect Students From Sexual Assault has established recommendations for colleges and universities to improve the response and prevention efforts in addressing sexual assault on campuses as a priority. The six core elements are:

1. Coordinated Campus and Community Response
2. Prevention and Education
3. Policy Development and Implementation
4. Reporting Options, Advocacy, and Support Services
5. Climate Surveys, Performance Measurement, and Evaluation
6. Transparency

In addition, the Title IX of the Education Amendments Act of 1972 is a federal civil rights law that requires schools receiving federal funding to prohibit sex discrimination in educational programs (DeMatteo, Galloway, Arnold, & Patel, 2015). Under this law, sexual violence is defined as a form of sex discrimination and protects all students from sexual violence. The law requires employees within the school system to respond appropriately to reports of sexual violence and to report such acts to appropriate school officials. It also requires training of employees, including their understanding of how to respond appropriately to reports of sexual violence. There is also an established method on how to respond and report sexual violence to the appropriate school officials.

SCHOOL NURSES

Nurses working in university healthcare centers may be the first to encounter victims of sexual assault. Nurses need to be aware of the risk factors associated with sexual assault, as students may first present for healthcare needs that are the result of a sexual assault. Educating college students in what constitutes sexual violence is an area that needs improvement. Students often do not know what a sexual assault actually is, so all students should be educated, as victims may not know that they have been assaulted and perpetrators may not know their actions constitute assault. Oftentimes, rape myths are believed by college students and reporting an assault or seeking help after an assault is not done, due to fear of no one believing them, self-blame, peer pressure, or being exiled from certain social circles (Hayes, Abbott, & Cooks, 2016; Navarro & Tewksbury, 2017). As such, educational efforts should be implemented to dispel rape myths. Lastly, educational programs aimed at students can help make college campuses free of sexual violence.

CONSENT

Another aspect of education for college students involves consent and what it correctly entails. "Consent" in the context of sexual assault refers to the ability to give approval freely to engage in sexual activities. Sexual violence, especially when the victim and perpetrator are under the influence of substances, may not always be possible to articulate. An inability to give consent can be due to a number of issues, such as age, mental status, intoxication, being unconscious, or sleeping. Sexual acts are performed when the individual is in a state in which there is an inability to give consent. Lastly, there may also be a context in which the individual is unable to refuse and this can be due to a number of circumstances, such as fear of physical violence or intimidation.

BYSTANDER INTERVENTION

Bystander intervention is a notable program designed to promote others in speaking out when there is a crime about to be committed or while one is being committed (Berkowitz, 2009). The emphasis is on a community response to a witnessed crime. The bystander is someone who is not involved in the crime and is a witness to the events that are happening and able to act by stopping or preventing the crime. In regards to sexual assault, this would entail intervention if there is a risk or actual incident witness of sexual harassment, sexual assault, dating violence, domestic violence, or stalking. There are four phases: noticing the event, interpreting it as a problem, feeling responsible to act, and having the necessary skills to act (NSVRC, 2018).

Fast Facts

The cardinal rule to bystander intervention is to act only if it is safe to do so.

TIPS ON BYSTANDER INTERVENTION

- Disrupt the situation. If noticing a crime being committed or someone at risk, you should disrupt what is happening or distract the perpetrator only if this is a safe option and does not put you at risk.
- Do not act alone; try to get other bystanders to help, or tell another friend what is going on.
- Confront the perpetrator and let the perpetator know that his or her behavior or actions are wrong.
- See yourself as being part of the solution; acknowledge you may have certain aspects or privileges that make it easier for you to speak up and be listened to.
- Educate yourself and others on what to do.
- Call 911.

CONCLUSION

Campus sexual assault is a serious problem that impacts the health and academics of college students. Having an understanding of the scope of the problem will enable forensic nurses and nurses who work with college students to acquire the necessary skills in treating and preventing campus sexual assault.

References

Berkowitz, A. (2009). *Response ability: A complete guide to bystander intervention.* Chicago, IL: Beck & Co.

Cantor, D., Fisher, B., Chibnall, S. H., Townsend, R., Lee, H., Thomas, G., Bruce, C., & Thomas, G. (2015). Report on the AAU Campus Climate Survey on Sexual Assault and Sexual Misconduct. Retrieved from https://www.aau.edu/sites/default/files/%40%20Files/Climate%20Survey/AAU_Campus_Climate_Survey_12_14_15.pdf

DeMatteo, D., Galloway, M., Arnold, S., & Patel, U. (2015). Sexual assault on college campuses: A 50-state survey of criminal sexual assault statutes and their relevance to campus sexual assault. *Psychology, Public Policy, and Law, 21*(3), 227–228. doi:10.1037/law0000055

Feit, N. (2017). Man posing as Uber driver held women against their will, police say. *Miami Herald.* Retrieved from http://www.miamiherald.com/news/local/crime/article188321529.html

Glaser, R. (2018). Student reports sexual battery by Lyft driver near dorms—The panther online. Retrieved from http://www.thepantheronline.com/news/student-reports-sexual-battery-lyft-driver-near-dorms

Hayes, R., Abbott, R., & Cook, S. (2016). It's her fault: Student acceptance of rape myths on two college campuses. *Violence Against Women, 22*(13), 1540–1555. doi:10.1177/1077801216630147

Krebs, C., Lindquist, C., Berzofsky, M., Shook-Sa, B., Peterson, K., Planty, M., . . . & Stroop, J. (2016). *Campus climate survey validation study: Final technical report.* Washington, DC: Bureau of Justice Statistics, U.S. Department of Justice. Retrieved from https://www.bjs.gov/content/pub/pdf/ccsvsftr.pdf

Lorenz, K., & Ullman, S. E. (2016). Alcohol and sexual assault victimization: Research findings and future directions. *Aggression and Violent Behavior, 31*, 82–94. doi:10.1016/j.avb.2016.08.001

National Sexual Violence Resource Center (NSVRC). (2018). Bystander intervention tips and strategies. Retrieved from https://www.nsvrc.org/bystander-intervention-tips-and-strategies

Navarro, J. C., & Tewksbury, R. (2017). National comparisons of rape myth acceptance predictors between nonathletes and athletes from multi-institutional settings. *Sexual Abuse.* Epub ahead of print September 1. doi:10.1177/1079063217732790

Nudd, T. (2017). Tostitos' new party bag knows when you've been drinking and will even call you an Uber. Retrieved from http://www.adweek.com/creativity/tostitos-new-party-bag-knows-when-youve-been-drinking-and-will-even-call-you-uber-175727

Roderick, L. (2016). Budweiser looks to more Uber tie-ups after responsible drinking ad. Retrieved from https://www.marketingweek.com/2016/12/07/budweiser-looks-uber-tie-ups

Sinozich, S., & Langton, L. (2014). *Rape and sexual assault victimization among college-age females, 1995–2013.* Washington, DC: U.S. Department of Justice. Retrieved from https://www.bjs.gov/content/pub/pdf/rsavcaf9513.pdf

Uber. (2017). Uber | MADD: Get home safe. Retrieved from https://www.uber.com/partner/madd

9

Interpersonal Violence

Meredith J. Scannell and Patricia A. Normandin

Interpersonal violence (IPV) is a major public health problem that occurs in all types of relationships: heterosexual, lesbian, gay, bisexual, and transgender. IPV is often referred to as "domestic violence," "intimate partner violence," or "battering." IPV is a pattern of assaultive and abusive behaviors in which power, control, and psychological and abusive behaviors are used within an intimate relationship, which threatens a person's well-being. Nurses in all settings may come in contact with survivors of IPV and therefore they must have an understanding of the scope of the problem and difficulties in exiting an IPV relationship so that violence does not escalate, and safety is paramount.

At the end of the chapter, the nurse will be able to:

1. Describe the scope of the problem of IPV.
2. Identify different types of abuse and how they may present in different individuals.
3. Understand patients vulnerable to IPV and how cultural backgrounds impact one's ability to seek help and leave an IPV situation.
4. List elements of a safety plan.

BACKGROUND

IPV occurs within groups of all ages, gender, socioeconomic status, religion, race, and ethnicity. The majority of IPV incidents are carried out by men and experienced by women. In the United States, 4.7 million women are physically assaulted each year. About 35.6% of women have experienced rape, physical violence, or stalking within an IPV relationship in their lifetimes (Black et al., 2011).

The intentionality of the violence is often described as a "wheel of violence" and is often cyclical in nature. The abuse that occurs does not happen all the time; it often occurs in a cyclical fashion, which is often unpredictable and over time increases in frequency and intensity (deBenedictis, Jaffe, & Segal, 2018). There are several different types of abuse that a perpetrator uses to maintain control; oftentimes the survivor experiences more than one type of abuse (Table 9.1).

Table 9.1

Types of Interpersonal Violence	
Type of Abuse	**Examples**
Physical abuse	Direct acts: slapping, punching, kicking, biting, strangulation, burns, attacking with weapon, throwing objects, depriving the partner of sleep Indirect acts: subjecting to reckless driving, withholding medical attention
Emotional abuse	Direct acts: name-calling, stalking, withholding affection, threatening to leave, publicly humiliating partner, convincing the partner he or she has mental health problems Indirect acts: breaking promises, playing mind games, unfaithful after promising to be monogamous
Economic abuse	Direct acts: controling all money, preventing partner from working, forcing partner to work excessively and taking all money Indirect acts: interfering with job, ruining credit ratings
Sexual abuse	Direct acts: forcing unwanted or humiliating sexual activity, forcing, coercing or manipulating sexual activity, forcing sexual activity with others Indirect acts: contraception/pregnancy coercion, withholding sex as punishment, publicly discussing sex life with survivor to others, infecting partner with sexually transmitted infections
Isolation	Direct acts: cutting partner off from friends and family; denying privacy; preventing from leaving the house; denying communication from other people; controlling social media, phone calls, and emails Indirect acts: calling constantly, disabling care, listening in on phone calls, setting up video recording

(continued)

Table 9.1

Types of Interpersonal Violence (*continued*)

Type of Abuse	Examples
Use of privilege	Direct acts: treating partner like a servant, name-calling in the form of racial or ethnic slurs, threatening immigration status, forcing religious beliefs on the partner, controlling what the partner wears Indirect acts: mistranslating information, encouraging others (family, friends) to engage in abusive activities towards the partner
Intimidation	Direct acts: making physical gestures of hitting or throwing things, displaying a weapon such as a knife or gun, destroying personal property: clothing, passport, driver's license Indirect acts: hurting pets
Use of children	Direct acts: threatening or punishing the children, forcing the children to watch physical and sexual violent acts Indirect acts: having the children to act as spies, using visitation of children as a method to have contact with the partner, punishing the partner for not having a baby of the desired sex, turning the children against the partner
Minimizing, denying, and blaming	Direct acts: denying acts of abuse, minimizing the seriousness of the abuse, refusing medical care Indirect acts: blaming the behavior on the partner, refusing to accept responsibility
Threats	Direct acts: threatening to harm the partner's family, friends, pets, property Indirect acts: Threatening to kill self or children

Source: Missouri Coalition Against Domestic and Sexual Violence. (2015). *Understanding the nature and dynamics of domestic violence.* Retrieved from https://www.mocadsv.org/FileStream.aspx?FileID=2; O'Campo, P., Smylie, J., Minh, A., Omand, M., & Cyriac, A. (2015). Conceptualizing acts and behaviours that comprise intimate partner violence: A concept map. *Health Expectations, 18*(6), 1968–1981. doi:10.1111/hex.12291

LESBIAN, GAY, BISEXUAL, TRANSGENDER, QUEER/QUESTIONING, AND INTERSEX PERSONS

The IPV statistics of lesbian, gay, bisexual, transgender, queer/questioning, and intersex (LGBTQI) persons demonstrate that they have equal to or higher IPV rates than heterosexual persons (NCADV, 2018). Rates of IPV among same-sex couples have been reported as high as 21.5% for men and 35.4% for women (Tjaden & Thoennes, 2000). These individuals face forms of IPV that are specific to the LGBTQI individuals, such as getting outed to family, friends, or coworkers regarding their sexual orientation or their gender identity or having private medical information disclosed such as HIV status. Calton et al. (2016) researched the unique issues LGBTQI individuals face regarding IPV and found women who are in an IPV relationship with other women may have difficulties in having outside individuals understand the severity of the abuse, in that others will view the abuse as a "cat fight" and not as IPV, and this results in fewer outside people wanting to get involved or offer help. Men who have sex with men too have unique challenges regarding IPV. Barriers exist for LGBTQI individuals in IPV situations in identification and availability of shelters that mean their individual needs. Individuals in the transgender communities may face challenges of being accepted into certain-gender-only shelters when they are in a transitioning period, or they may be turned away because of not being the right gender. Laws in some states may not recognize same-sex partners; therefore they may not grant protective orders. These laws and other discriminatory or lack of LGBTQI policies, practices, and resources impact individuals from seeking and accessing services.

IMMIGRANT POPULATIONS

Immigrants are an understudied population in terms of IPV, often due to cultural and language barriers. IPV is highly prevalent among immigrants and actual numbers are often hard to determine. A large systematic review of immigrant populations in the United States found rates of IPV to range from 15.5% to 70%, with the highest rates of IPV found within the South Asian and Hispanic communities (Breiding et al., 2014). Cultural values and beliefs shape how IPV is viewed, experienced, and tolerated in different populations. Some cultures do

BOX 9.1   CULTURAL CONCERNS REGARDING IPV

- Language barriers
- Impact of community and family reaction
- Religious beliefs, unable to separate or divorce
- Belief of need to be submissive
- Fear of law enforcement
- Isolation from family, friends

- Lack of understanding about IPV
- Fear of ostracization from family
- Shame/stigma in discussing with family
- Male dominance is norm
- Fear of deportation
- Fear of abuser being deported

not identify domestic values or may have beliefs that it is an actual right of the husband within a marriage for the female to be submissive to her husband, or the family may be influencing them to stay.

Access to services may be severely impacted due to several cultural barriers. For one, the individual may be isolated and not allowed to learn the language of the country of immigration and be unaware of services or how to access them. There is also an underlying fear of law enforcement officials or other individuals with authority, and therefore IPV survivors may not want to come forward. Immigration status can also be a barrier in seeking help, with the fear of the survivor, children, or abuser being deported.

The impact of domestic violence can have a significant effect on the physical and mental health of individuals (Ingemann-Hansen & Charles, 2013). See Table 9.2 Acute and long-term effects of abuse that occur in different IPV situations. Anytime a survivor presents to a healthcare center after an IPV relationship or after an acute traumatic abuse, the survivor should be treated for all life-threatening injuries (Ingemann-Hansen & Charles, 2013). Given the degree of impact that IPV can have on health, a complete health assessment and head-to-toe exam should be performed.

Table 9.2

Acute and Long-term Effects of Abuse

Type of Abuse	Acute Effect	Long-Term Effect
Physical abuse	■ Injuries: cuts, lacerations, bruises, fractures ■ Defensive injuries: wounds sustained while protecting oneself ■ Asthma ■ Bladder and kidney infections ■ Headaches ■ Strangulation; loss of memory, subconjunctival hemorrhage, sore throat, difficulty swallowing, respiratory distress, cardiac arrythmias ■ Permanent disabilities ■ Death	■ Asthma ■ Bladder and kidney infections ■ Circulatory conditions ■ Cardiovascular disease ■ Fibromyalgia ■ Irritable bowel syndrome ■ Chronic pain syndromes ■ Central nervous system disorders ■ Gastrointestinal disorders ■ Joint disease ■ Migraines and headaches ■ Old fractures, untreated and unhealed ■ Behavioral changes; smoking, substance abuse

(continued)

Table 9.2

Acute and Long-term Effects of Abuse (*continued*)

Type of Abuse	Acute Effect	Long-Term Effect
Sexual abuse	■ Sexually transmitted infections, including HIV/AIDS ■ Unintended pregnancy	■ Sexual dysfunction ■ Gynecological disorders ■ Delayed prenatal care ■ Preterm delivery ■ Pregnancy difficulties like low birth weight babies and perinatal deaths
Physiological abuse	■ Anxiety ■ Antisocial behavior ■ Suicidal behavior in females ■ Sleep disturbances ■ Flashbacks ■ Replaying assault in the mind	■ Depression ■ Symptoms of posttraumatic stress disorder (PTSD) ■ Low self-esteem ■ Inability to trust others, especially in intimate relationships ■ Fear of intimacy ■ Emotional detachment
Health effects during pregnancy	■ Placental abruption ■ Inadequate prenatal care ■ Anemia ■ Kidney infections ■ Miscarriage ■ Preterm labor ■ Increased risk for C-section ■ Still birth ■ Low birth weight/ intrauterine growth restriction ■ Perinatal fetal distress ■ Fetal or neonatal death	

One red flag of IPV is the degree of injuries a survivor sustains in the course of an IPV relationship. When suspecting or documenting cases of IPV, it is essential to document injuries accurately. Injuries can present at different time periods after an assault, and although injuries may have been present at an earlier evaluation, newer injuries could now be showing. Additionally, old injuries should be examined for stages of healing. If someone is in a relationship with ongoing violence or assaults, then there may be bruising and injuries in many different stages of healing.

Fast Facts

The BALD STEP mnemonic is one assessment tool that focuses on trauma-related injuries and allows for more precise documentation of general and genital injuries. The BALD STEP covers specific trauma-related injuries: B—bite mark, bleeding, bruise, burn; A—abrasion, avulsion; L—laceration; D—deformity; S—swelling, stains; T—tenderness, trace evidence; E—erythema; P—patterns, petechiae, penetrating wounds (Carter-Snell, 2011).

There can be many varying injuries and in different stages of healing, reflected in the different colors in bruising. Bite mark is a common injury, which can leave a mark from the actual bite or mark from suction that was applied with the bite. There may be defensive wounds found on the backs of arms with the women trying to defend themselves. Documenting exam findings should be accurate, thorough, and precise. All injuries should be documented utilizing medicolegal terminology even if photographs were taken. Follow your agency and jurisdiction guidelines for the use of forensic photographs. A body diagram map should be used for documenting injuries and foreign bodies to demonstrate where on the body they occurred. Nurses should do a systematic head-to-toe assessment to document injuries. Documentation should include size, depth, shape, and pattern of the injury and measurements if possible according to the BALD STEP mnemonic (Carter-Snell, 2011).

SCREENING

All patients who present for care in any healthcare setting should be universally screened for IPV (Normandin, 2015). Forensic nurses are in an ideal situation to be able to identify cases of IPV and make necessary referrals and help patients to develop strategies to keep them safe. Incorporate therapeutic communication that is respectful and caring and a trauma-informed approach and interventions (U.S. Department of Health and Human Services, 2018).

BEST PRACTICE SCREENING STRATEGIES TO IDENTIFY SIGNS AND SYMPTOMS OF IPV

- Utilize safety screening tools identified by your agency.
- Screen all patients privately.
- Screen all patients regardless of age, gender, or financial/economic situation.
- Identify individual barriers to screening.

- Develop individual strategies to overcome barriers to screening.
- Screen for safety when the survivor is alone.
- Communicate in a caring manner.
- Approach each patient from a trauma-informed framework (U.S. Department of Health and Human Services, 2018).
- Screen all mothers who bring their children or themselves for vague emergency complaints because research has shown IPV survivors have a higher healthcare services utilization (Correa, 2018; Normandin, 2015).
- Mothers of children older than 3 years should be screened separately from their child, because of the possibility of the child hearing the questions and mother's answers and reporting back to the perpetrator (Normandin, 2015).
- Each agency needs policies and procedures in screening/treatment of survivors of violence/neglect.
- Follow your agency's policies and procedures in screening/treatment of survivors of violence/neglect.
- Healthcare administrators and educators need to ensure training and individual healthcare provider's self-efficacy in screening for violence/neglect.

LEAVING AN IPV SITUATION

Leaving an IPV relationship is often a complex and dangerous time for the survivor, and may take several attempts before someone in an IPV is successfully able to leave. The survivor may be fearful of retaliation. Due to the complex nature of IPV, survivors often have job instability, bad credit, and little housing track record, making their ability to afford and obtain independent housing difficult. In addition, the survivor may be relying on social services, and options for housing may include long wait times, substandard housing arrangements, or housing in unsafe neighborhoods. The survivor may have to weigh different choices such as protecting the children from unsafe or substandard housing, or leaving and risk losing the children due to custody issues. Furthermore, survivors may lack the economic means or may be dependent on the batterer. They are often hopeful that the partner will change, so they stay and endure further violence.

Most individuals in an IPV relationship will leave and return several times to the abuser before permanently separating from the batterer. Leaving must be done in a trauma-informed approach, which empowers the survivors, recognizes their goals, and does not further jeopardize their safety. It is critical to empower an individual to develop a safety plan to implement when in an IPV relationship. A safety plan is a survivor's strategy to reduce the risk of leaving an IPV relationship. A lethality risk assessment should be conducted with the individual to review potential dangers and help them develop a safety plan with support services.

ELEMENTS IN A SAFETY PLAN

- Plan a safe place to which to go when in danger; avoid rooms with weapons (e.g., kitchen)
- Identify support persons—family, friends, and neighbors who can assist in an emergency
- Keep your cell phone close by
- Have a method or code to contact your support person when danger is occurring or imminent
- Have a plan for leaving in an emergency with essential items in a safe and easily accessible place, such as a small bag packed with important documents, cash, passports, birth certificates, identification, legal documents, spare keys, extra clothing, and prescriptions
- Initiate contacts to resources that can help with legal or various social service applications and restraining orders
- Identify economic, legal, and educational resources
- Educate children in calling 911, avoiding danger
- Receive education on technology safety, Internet, text messages, Global Positioning System (GPS) tracking, computer monitoring

Resources IPV survivors may need include:

- Survivor-focused recovery programs
- Trauma counselors
- Support groups, helplines, and drop-in services
- Financial empowerment programs
- Family Justice programs
- Parenting After Violence classes
- Rape crisis centers
- Restraining orders
- Immigration legal services
- Legal services for any outstanding charges due to IPV situations, which may have resulted in assault or felony charges against the IPV survivor
- Provide family legal services if the IPV survivor has minor children, to assist in legal family matters
- Shelter if the IPV survivor is homeless
- If the survivor is both in an IPV and human trafficking situation, he or she may have different legal service needs

- If homeless and IPV and human trafficking survivor, a shelter that accommodates all those situations is ideal
- Legal services for the IPV survivor who is also in a human trafficking situation may require immigration legal services and other legal services related to their personal situation

CONCLUSION

IPV remains a complex public health problem that impacts individuals, families, and communities. Having an understanding of the scope of the complexities of the types of violence and those at risk allows for nurses to help provide care, support, and resources in a manner that promotes safety. Nurses in all healthcare settings can be instrumental in identifying patients at risk as well as those in current unsafe situations. With a better understanding of necessary information regarding IPV and essential safety aspects, nurses will be able to help patients while minimizing any risk to them, enabling patients to become empowered.

RESOURCES

National Coalition Against Domestic Violence: https://ncadv.org, 2018

References

Black, M. C., Basile, K. C., Breiding, M. J., Smith, S. G., Walters, M. L., Merrick, M. T., . . . Stevens, M. R. (2011). *The national intimate partner and sexual violence survey (NISVS): 2010 summary report*. Atlanta, GA: National Center for Injury Prevention and Control, Centers for Disease Control and Prevention.

Breiding, M., Smith, S., Basile, K., Walters, M., Chen, J., and Merrick, M. (2014). Prevalence and characteristics of sexual violence, stalking, and intimate partner violence victimization: National Intimate Partner and Sexual Violence Survey, United States, 2011. *Morbidity and Mortality Weekly Report, 63*(SS08), 1–18. Retrieved from https://www.cdc.gov/mmwr/preview/mmwrhtml/ss6308a1.htm

Calton, J. M., Lauren, B. C., & Gebhard, K. T. (2016). Barriers to help seeking for lesbian, gay, bisexual, transgender, and queer survivors of intimate partner violence. *Trauma, Violence, & Abuse, 17*(5), 585–600. doi:10.1177/1524838015585318

Carter-Snell, C. (2011). Injury documentation: Using the BALD STEP mnemonic and the RCMP sexual assault kit. *Outlook, 34*(1), 15–20.

Correa, N. P. (2018, January). An assessment of screening for intimate partner violence. Texas Children's Hospital, Department of Pediatrics, Baylor College of Medicine, Adverse Childhood Experiences Coalition-Intimate Partner Violence Workgroup. Retrieved from https://www.texaschildrens.org/sites/default/files/uploads/IPV%20Assessment%20.Final.pdf

deBenedictis, T., Jaffe, J., & Segal, J. (2018). Domestic violence and abuse: Types, signs, symptoms, causes, and effects. *American Academy of Experts in Traumatic Stress.* Retrieved from http://www.aaets.org/article144.htm

Ingemann-Hansen, O., & Charles, A. V. (2013). Forensic medical examination of adolescent and adult victims of sexual violence. *Best Practice & Research Clinical Obstetrics & Gynaecology, 27*(1), 91–102. doi:10.1016/j.bpobgyn.2012.08.014

Missouri Coalition Against Domestic and Sexual Violence. (2015). *Understanding the nature and dynamics of domestic violence.* Retrieved from https://www.mocadsv.org/FileStream.aspx?FileID=2

National Coalition Against Domestic Violence (NCADV). (2018). Retrieved from https://ncadv.org

Normandin, P. A. (2015). Identifying maternal intimate partner violence in the emergency department. *Journal of Emergency Nursing, 41*(5), 444–446. doi:10.1016/j.jen.2015.05.011

O'Campo, P., Smylie, J., Minh, A., Omand, M., & Cyriac, A. (2015). Conceptualizing acts and behaviours that comprise intimate partner violence: A concept map. *Health Expectations, 18*(6), 1968–1981. doi:10.1111/hex.12291

Statistics. (2018). The National Domestic Violence Hotline. Retrieved from https://www.thehotline.org/resources/statistics/

Tjaden, P. G., & Thoennes, N. (2000). *Extent, nature, and consequences of intimate partner violence.* Washington, DC: Department of Justice (US).

U.S. Department of Health and Human Services. (2018). Trauma-informed approach and trauma-specific interventions. *Substance Abuse and Mental Health Services Administration.* Retrieved from https://www.samhsa.gov/nctic/trauma-interventions

III

Age-Related Violence

10

Child Maltreatment

Kristine Ruggiero

Child abuse and neglect are serious public health problems in the United States. For example, each year, 2 million children are seriously abused. At least 1,000 of these children die as a result of their injuries. The World Health Organization (WHO, 1999) Consultation on Child Abuse Prevention drafted the following definition: "Child abuse or maltreatment constitutes all forms of physical and/or emotional ill-treatment, sexual abuse, neglect or negligent treatment or commercial or other exploitation, resulting in actual or potential harm to the child's health, survival, development or dignity in the context of a relationship of responsibility, trust or power" (p. 16). This definition covers a broad spectrum of abuse. This chapter focuses on the forensic nurse's role in evaluation of suspected child abuse and neglect.

At the end of this chapter, the nurse will be able to:

1. State the various types of child maltreatment.
2. Describe the nurse's role as a mandated reporter in cases of suspected child abuse and neglect.
3. List three "red flag" findings for suspected abuse and neglect.
4. Describe how a forensic interview is conducted in cases where child abuse and/or neglect are suspected.
5. List three ways a forensic nurse can address suspected child maltreatment in a culturally sensitive manner.

BACKGROUND

The forensic nurse caring for children at risk for abuse and neglect needs to recognize the different types of child maltreatment and understand his or her role in the workup of suspected abuse and neglect. The assessment as outlined by obtaining a history and physical examination is also discussed. The role of the forensic nurse may encompass reporting suspected abuse; assessing the consistency of the explanation, the child's developmental capabilities, and the characteristics of the injury or injuries; and coordinating with other professionals to provide immediate and long-term treatment and follow-up for victims.

TYPES OF CHILD ABUSE AND NEGLECT

Child physical abuse affects children of all ages, genders, ethnicities, and socioeconomic groups. Male and female children experience similar rates of physical abuse. There are five types of child maltreatment (discussed in the following list). The four major forms of child maltreatment are physical abuse, sexual abuse, emotional abuse, and neglect; often abandonment is captured under neglect. Despite the subtle state-to-state differences in what constitutes child maltreatment, the following is a summary of historically agreed upon terminology and classification:

1. Physical abuse means the nonaccidental infliction of physical injury on a child, and it includes:
   a. Striking or hitting a child with a closed fist
   b. Interfering with a child's breathing
2. Sexual abuse means either committing or allowing any sexual offense against a child as defined in criminal codes, and it includes:
   a. Intentionally touching, either directly or through the clothing, the sexual or other intimate parts of a child
   b. Allowing or causing a child to engage in touching the sexual or other intimate parts of another for sexual gratification of the person responsible for the child, the child, or a third party
3. Sexual exploitation means allowing or causing a child to engage in:
   a. Prostitution
   b. Sexually explicit, obscene, or pornographic activity to be photographed, filmed, or electronically reproduced or transmitted

Fast Facts

Knowing the different types of child abuse is necessary so that it can be identified early.

   c. Sexually explicit, obscene, or pornographic activity as part of a live performance or for the benefit of sexual gratification of another person

4. Child maltreatment or negligent treatment:

   a. An act of failure to act or a pattern of inaction that shows a serious disregard of consequences and constitutes a clear and present danger to a child's health, welfare, or safety. Neglect includes (but is not limited to) failure to provide adequate food, shelter, clothing, supervision, or healthcare necessary for a child's health, welfare, or safety.

   b. Poverty and/or homelessness do not constitute neglect in and of themselves as well as actions and failures to act that result in injury or that cause a substantial risk of injury to the physical, emotional, and/or cognitive development of a child.

5. Abandonment means the parent deserts the child with an intent to abandon or leaves the child without necessities of life, such as food, water, or shelter, or forgoes parental rights, functions, duties, and obligations for extended periods of time:

   a. The exception to this type of child maltreatment is if a newborn is abandoned at a hospital, fire station, or another designated health clinic. The Safety of Newborn Children Act was enacted to ensure that abandonment does not happen and that all newborns have the opportunity for a stable home life. This act allows a parent to transfer a newborn anonymously and without criminal liability.

To access the statutes for a specific state or territory, visit the state statutes search of the Child Welfare Information Gateway at www.childwelfare.gov/topics/systemwide/laws-policies/state (Child Welfare Information Gateway, 2016).

IMPACT OF CHILD ABUSE AND NEGLECT

The impact and consequences of child abuse and neglect can be lifelong on victims' well-being. Children who have experienced the trauma of abuse or neglect are at risk of experiencing cognitive delays, emotional difficulties, and other issues.

MANDATED REPORTING: WHO REPORTS?

Mandatory reporting refers to a legal obligation to report certain kinds of concern to child-welfare authorities. Overall, children rarely disclose their own suffering, and because perpetrators of child abuse and neglect are often unlikely to reveal this to authorities, the intent of mandatory reporting is to encourage the good faith reporting of concerns for children to protect them. Since children who are being abused and neglected are oftentimes unable to verbalize and advocate for themselves, mandated reporters are charged with recognizing the signs and symptoms of child maltreatment so that children can be protected from harm. As such, the real annual incidence of child abuse and neglect far exceeds the number of cases that are brought to the attention of welfare agencies.

A mandatory reporting law is a statutory duty to report suspected cases of designated types of child maltreatment to child-welfare agencies. Most states have regulations regarding mandatory reporting of suspected child abuse and neglect. In some jurisdictions, the duty is imposed on all citizens. In other areas, the duty to report is placed on certain occupations, specifically those most likely to encounter children during their work. Nurses are mandated reporters. Other examples of mandated reporters include teachers, clinicians, school counselors, therapists, police officers, coroners, child care providers, and Department of Corrections personnel. Information on specific state laws are provided by the Children's Bureau (Administration for Children and Families, U.S. Department of Health and Human Services); for a complete list of mandated reporters in each state, see www.childwelfare.gov/topics/systemwide/ laws-policies/state.

Fast Facts

Most nurses are considered mandatory reporters for suspicion of any forms of child abuse; failure to do so could result in legal and board-of-nursing penalties.

MANDATED REPORTING: WHAT IS MY OBLIGATION?

Mandated reporters must report suspected child abuse or neglect (or cause a report to be made) to law enforcement or Child Protection Services (CPS) when they believe a child has suffered abuse or neglect or may be at risk for abuse or neglect. CPS is part of the juvenile system, which is charged with protecting the child, and the criminal justice system prosecutes any crimes committed. This report must be made at the first opportunity and no later than 48 hours after suspected abuse or neglect has occurred. Mandated reporters' failure to report known or suspected child abuse and neglect may be guilty of a gross misdemeanor. Table 10.1 lists possible red flags that either a child or a parent or a caretaker may be exhibiting in which child abuse may be suspected.

MANDATED REPORTING: WHOM TO CONTACT?

- Your local police station
- Your local CPS agency

- National Child Abuse Hotline: 1-800-4-A-Child
- Hotlines for each state: www.childwelfare.gov/pubs/reslist/rl_dsp. cfm?rs_id=5&rate_chno=W-00082

CHILDREN AT RISK FOR CHILD ABUSE AND NEGLECT

BOX 10.1 CHARACTERISTICS OF THE CHILD AT RISK FOR CHILD ABUSE AND NEGLECT

- Infants and young children (<3 years)
- Children with mental or physical disabilities
- Children with older siblings
- The "challenging" child
- Children in dysfunctional or isolated families
- Children where there is substance abuse in the home
- Unrealistic parental expectations

Table 10.1

Red Flag Findings for Possible Child Abuse and Neglect

Possible Signs of Child Maltreatment (Child)	Possible Signs of Child Maltreatment by Parent/Caretaker
■ Shows sudden changes in behavior or school performance	■ Lack of concern for child's injuries/pain
■ Has learning problems that cannot be attributed to specific physical or psychological causes	■ Inability/unwillingness to comfort child
■ Is always watchful, as though preparing for something bad to happen	■ Delay in seeking needed medical care
■ Lacks adult supervision	■ Incompatible or absent history
■ Is overly compliant, passive, or withdrawn	■ Refusal to be separated from child for purpose of obtaining separate histories
■ Comes to school or other activities early, stays late, and does not want to go home	■ History of substance abuse by any caregivers or people living in the home
■ Has not received help for physical or medical problems brought to the parent's attention	■ Social and financial stressors

The forensic nurse's role in detecting suspicious injuries and reporting of abuse can prevent further abusive trauma and can facilitate appropriate evaluation, referral, investigation, and outcomes for these children and families. There follow strategies for successful evaluation of suspected child abuse and neglect.

KEYS TO INTERVIEWING STRATEGIES FOR A FORENSIC NURSE WHEN INTERVIEWING A PARENT/CAREGIVER SUSPECTED OF ABUSE AND NEGLECT

- Remain objective.
- Ask open-ended questions to parent/caretaker.
- If the child is verbal, consider separating the child and parent/caregiver to obtain separate detailed histories (noting any discrepancies between the two).
- Gather information in a nonaccusatory but detailed manner.

WORKUP OF SUSPECTED CHILD ABUSE AND NEGLECT

- History
    - The evidence collection process begins with taking a thorough history.
        - Note how the injuries were sustained and relevant medical conditions that the patient may have (e.g., bleeding disorders, Ricketts, vitamin deficiencies, musculoskeletal conditions).
        - The nurse should record/document all findings exactly as they are said (using quotation marks for verbatim responses), and use objective language; also, document any intervention(s) taken.
        - Include other areas of physical or mental concern that may relate to the abuse:
            - Past medical history (including trauma, hospitalizations, congenital conditions, chronic illnesses)
            - Family history (including bleeding, bone disorders, and metabolic or genetic disorders)
            - Pregnancy history (including wanted/unwanted, planned/unplanned, prenatal care, postnatal complications, postpartum depression, delivery in nonhospital settings)
            - Family patterns of discipline
            - History of past abuse to the child or siblings
- Social evaluation
    - Risk factors including dysfunctional family and substance abuse in the home
    - Handicapped, premature, or young child (<3 years)

- Complete physical examination
  - Note if the history appears consistent with the injury and developmental abilities of the child.
    - Does the history match up with the physical exam findings (e.g., if the baby rolled from a couch and now has retinal hemorrhaging)?
  - Obtain photographs and/or body diagrams and measurements of suspected abuse and neglect.
    - Photography: Many states do not require parental consent to document injuries of suspected abuse and neglect. Use a Polaroid or digital camera to take images. Note the location, size, shape, color, and apparent age of any markings/ burns/bruising. Also, include anatomical charts and color photographs of the injuries before treatment (if possible).
    - One photograph should be a full body shot that includes the victim's face. This clearly links the injuries to the victim.
    - Photographs should never be used as a substitute for accurate and thorough medical documentation.
    - Measurements describing markings should be made in centimeters and described according to size, shape, appearance, and location using a readily recognized landmark.
    - Note the patient's name and medical record number (MRN) on the back of the photograph.

Fast Facts

Different cultures may have different practices that can mimic some forms of child abuse; it is essential to understand the cultural background of the patient so that you can identify between a normal cultural practice and that of child abuse.

CULTURAL ASPECTS OF CHILD MALTREATMENT: WAYS THE FORENSIC NURSE CAN ADDRESS CHILD MALTREATMENT IN A CULTURALLY SENSITIVE MANNER

As a multicultural society, the relationship and influence of these diverse cultures to the understanding and identification of child abuse and neglect are challenging and complex (Killion, 2017). Forensic nurses who work with children are trained to deal with suspected child maltreatment; however they are challenged with providing culturally competent care. Often forensic nurses find themselves with the challenge of exploring and resolving the tension between definitions of harm in child protection practice and various cultural and child-rearing practices. We now outline important cultural considerations when approaching and dealing with the suspicion of child maltreatment, including identifying common barriers in working with children and families from culturally diverse backgrounds.

Cultural variation in what is considered "abuse" is a major reason child maltreatment can often be underreported and an often-undetected problem. Many cultural healing practices can mimic signs or symptoms of abuse. For example, certain cultural practices, such as coining (caogio), cupping (hijama), moxibustion, or a range of strategies to treat sunken or fallen fontanels (caida de mollera), may have physical manifestations that often mimic child abuse (Killion, 2017). Other cultural practices, specifically female genital mutilation/circumcision (FGM/C), which is a practice of mutilating or circumcising female genital organs, is against the law to perform in the United States (www.uscig.gov/humanitarian/victims-human-trafficking). The nurse's role in recognizing suspected child abuse includes appreciating that there are certain cultural healing practices that can mimic child abuse. The nurse should remain objective, obtain a detailed history, acknowledge the family's cultural healing practices, and be sensitive to these practices and rituals.

In addition to cultural healing practices, religious practice can imitate child neglect if a parent does not provide medical treatment for a child based on their religious beliefs. This is not considered child abuse or neglect; however, a court can order medical services or nonmedical services to a child if the child's health requires it. For example, when a child's parents are Jehovah's Witnesses and do not believe in blood transfusions but the child medically requires a blood transfusion, the court can intervene on the child's behalf and potentially require this.

CONCLUSION

Child abuse has significant long-term sequelae, including medical and mental health morbidity. Child physical abuse is a common problem of childhood. The forensic nurse is well positioned to recognize suspicious injuries and conduct a comprehensive history and physical examination in a culturally sensitive manner. Forensic nurses are uniquely qualified to work with patients, parents, and the family to evaluate suspected child maltreatment as well as work to prevent further abuse by linking the family with other resources and providing anticipatory guidance around normal child behavior and its management to patients and families at risk for child abuse and neglect.

References

Child Welfare Information Gateway. (2016). *Definitions of child abuse and neglect*. Washington, DC: U.S. Department of Health and Human Services, Children's Bureau.

Killion, C. M. (2017). Cultural healing practices that mimic child abuse. *Annals of Forensic Research*, 4(2), 1042.

World Health Organization. (1999). *Report of the consultation on child abuse prevention*, WHO, Geneva, 29–31 March 1999. Geneva, Switzerland: Author. Retrieved from http://www.who.int/iris/handle/10665/65900

11

Elder Maltreatment

Stacy Brady

Elder maltreatment is an increasingly serious issue worldwide, due mostly to the rise in the older adult population. Abuse of the elderly can happen to anyone and varies with culture. Signs and symptoms can sometimes mimic medical conditions, so being vigilant and asking about abuse during every interaction can help the elderly individual get the treatment or resources he or she needs. Nurses are mandatory reporters, so it is crucial to know your organization's policy and your state laws.

At the end of the chapter, the nurse will be able to:

1. Define elderly abuse.
2. Differentiate between the different types of elderly abuse.
3. Recognize the "red flags" of elderly abuse.
4. Explain elderly abuse reporting.
5. Identify various resources for elderly abuse.

BACKGROUND

Maltreatment of older people, commonly referred to as "elder abuse" or "elder mistreatment," was first labeled in a British scientific journal by Baker in 1975 under the term "granny battering." Baker's article started raising awareness of this growing issue, causing the United Kingdom and the United States to initiate research into abuse of the elderly, but each country had different views on the matter. The UK focused more on abuse in medical or institutional settings, while the United States viewed this as a family and domestic violence problem. Even though mistreatment of the elderly was first recognized in developed countries, there are reports and anecdotal evidence that this is a concern in developing countries all over the world. It is a multidimensional phenomenon and an international public health concern, urgently requiring the attention of all healthcare organizations, legislators, social welfare agencies, and communities (Chalise, 2017; Faircloth, 2016).

Maltreatment of the elderly is predicted to increase in many countries due to a rapidly aging population whose needs may not be fully met due to resource constraints. In 2015, the World Health Organization (WHO, 2018) reported a global population of 900 million people aged 60 or over and predicted this will more than double to about 2 billion people in 2050.

Abuse of the elderly is one of the most unrecognized and underreported social issues today. Approximately one in six people older than 60 years reported some form of abuse in the past year. This is likely to be miscalculated because a study in New York found only one in 24 cases of elderly abuse was actually reported (WHO, 2018). Therefore, any prevalence rates are likely to be underestimated. Furthermore, the defining age of an elderly individual differs between organizations, as some states define it as greater than 60 and others states greater than 65.

Different definitions have been found for elderly abuse, but in 2002 a more widely accepted definition was created by WHO and the International Network for the Prevention of Elder Abuse (INPEA). They defined elder abuse as "a single or repeated act, or lack of appropriate action, occurring within any relationship where there is an expectation of trust, which causes harm or distress to an older person" (Faircloth, 2016, p. 10). The definition implies that abuse occurs when there is some sort of trusting relationship between the older person and the abuser. The relationship could be as simple as a salesperson or as complex as a family member, such as a spouse or adult child, which occurs in 90% of abuse cases. There are also cultural variations regarding abuse of the elderly (Table 11.1; Leahy & Rosof-Williams, 2012; Pillemer, Burnes, Riffin, & Lachs, 2016).

Fast Facts

Elder abuse happens in all educational, racial, socioeconomic, family, religious, and cultural groups and appears in every setting: home, nursing home, institutions, and so on. Healthcare professionals working with diverse elders in potentially abusive relationships need to be sensitive to cultural differences so the interventions will be appropriate.

Table 11.1

Differences in Cultures

Latino

- Women expected to tolerate abuse and serve others
- Men expected to neglect self to care for others
- The need to protect family from shame
- Feelings of guilt if unable to provide care for elders at home
- Does not consider financial abuse true abuse

Chinese

- Family secret or private family matter
- Disrespect is considered worst form of abuse–being ignored and not invited to family gatherings
- Young population and the older population have cultural variations
- Isolation is common; kept from resources, programs, and services

Asian/Pacific Islander

- Uses the term "sacrifice" or "suffering" instead of abuse
- Emotional abuse is the most common and considered the worst
- Believe in filial piety
- Not acceptable to express emotions
- A representation of strength and honor is the ability to tolerate violence
- Verbal expression of emotion is not typical to outsiders

Japanese

- Emotional abuse is the worst form of abuse: intentionally not speaking to someone
- The perpetrator is usually the daughter-in-law
- Not caring for the elder is considered a lack of disrespect
- Considered a family secret and if exposed the person is considered a "traitor"
- Abuse should be tolerated in a passive manner; suffering quietly is common

Vietnamese

- Neglect is the worst form and shames the family
- Emotional abuse is the worst and most common form of abuse
- Kept in the family
- "Silent treatment" is extreme punishment
- Do not openly express feelings, but instead complain of physical symptoms

Native Americans

- Spiritual abuse is considered the most important: not being invited to ceremonies
- Denied access to healers

Arabic

- Women have limitations in freedom
- Financial abuse mostly performed by adult children
- Outside family caretaker rarely involved in any form of abuse
- Abuse is a private family affair

(continued)

Table 11.1

Differences in Cultures (*continued*)

Korean
- Financial exploitation is not considered a form of abuse; transferring money and property to the eldest son is the norm
- Neglect is considered okay and has a high tolerance
- Filial piety is emphasized, so long-term-care placement is a form of abuse

Asian Indian
- Eldest son has all the financial responsibilities
- Elder abandonment is considered when children leave home
- Physical abuse is uncommon

TYPES OF ABUSE

The first sign that further evaluation is needed is if the medical history is inconsistent or constantly changing, the patient discloses abuse, or the perpetrator will not leave the victim alone with the healthcare provider (Jett, 2016; Leahy & Rosof-Williams, 2012). Always ask the older adult if he or she is safe or feels threatened at any time during every interaction. The National Center of Elder Abuse (NCEA) stated that there are seven types of abuse of older adults: physical abuse, sexual abuse, neglect, self-neglect, emotional or psychological abuse, abandonment, and financial or material exploitation abuse. Know that elders may experience different types of abuse at the same time.

1. Physical abuse: The use of physical force that may or may not result in bodily harm, physical pain, or ongoing impairment. Examples of physical abuse could be the use of hands or objects to strike, beat, shove, bite, push, slap, shake, kick, or burn an elderly individual. It can also include using medication inappropriately, threatening with physical punishment, force feeding, or using restraints.

   Signs and symptoms of physical abuse:

   - Bruising: cannot be dated based on the bruise color. Bruises that occur at the same time can have a variation of different colors. Intentional bruising tends to be on the chest wall, abdomen, and more on softer areas of the body—thighs, cheeks, buttocks—and accidentals occur more on prominent bony areas
   - Fractures inconsistent with functional ability

- Welts; bite marks; rope/cord marks around ankles, wrists, or neck indicating restraints; burns; unexplained cuts/lacerations
- Delay in seeking care
- Broken glasses
- Sudden changes in personality or behavior
- Sprains, dislocations
- Patterns of injury: defensive wounds to hands, forearms, or soles of feet
- Injuries seen on well-protected body surfaces
- Injury unlikely given the patient's capabilities and history provided or no explanation given
- Multiple injuries in various stages of healing

2. Sexual abuse: Any nonconsensual sex or sexual contact with an elderly individual, including those who are unable to give consent.

BOX 11.1 PATTERNED BRUISES

Fingertip bruising: shaking/squeezing injury, often seen on face, neck, and extremities. Four oval/circular marks and/or a thumbprint. Example would be grasping an arm.

Pinch mark: two adjacent oval/round bruises the size of a fingertip or knuckle and may see fingernail marks outlining a clamshell arrangement of bruising.

Tramline/tram track: linear objects (flexible or rigid), lines of petechiae format the edges of contact, and if the object is flexible, it will wrap around the body and form a curved mark. The skin may be cut from the edge of the object. If the object is rigid, it will form a straight line resembling a "railroad track" and dips in the body will cause a break in the continuity of the mark.

Slap marks: fingermark imprints with bruising between the fingers and sparing where digits impact body.

Ligatures: bruises reflecting compression or constriction, circumferential or partly circumferential on limbs or neck. Bruising reveals the texture and size of the object.

Loop marks: could be caused by belt or extension cord. Narrow-spaced "tram tracks" forming a loop with central sparing and it is common for the tip of the loop to leave a cut or abrasion on the skin (Maryland Department of Health, 2008; Tully, 2015).

BOX 11.2 FINDINGS ASSOCIATED WITH INJURIES

Abrasion: partial or full-thickness wound where the skin is removed and debris may be embedded. It is caused by friction of the skin against a surface, such as a fall or bicycle crash. This can commonly be called a "scrape."

Avulsion: full-thickness wound where the skin and/or soft tissue has been torn away by blunt or shear force. Debris may be trapped in the injury.

Contusion: closed wound where a ruptured blood vessel leaks into surrounding tissue.

Hematoma: blood leaks under the skin and forms a palpable mass, which is a blood clot.

Laceration: open wounds from tearing or splitting of tissue through the dermis and epidermis from blunt or shearing forces. Also, could involve the underlying structures, such as tendons, muscles, organs, or ligaments.

Petechiae: small, nonraised reddish, purplish hemorrhagic dots. This is found with a variety of medical conditions and strangulation.

Puncture wounds: penetration of an object into the tissues. These can be superficial, such as being stuck with a needle, or a deeper injury, such as a stab wound.

Traumatic alopecia: traumatic loss of hair that could be associated with having hair pulled (Emergency Nurses Association, 2014; Leahy & Rosof-Williams, 2012).

This can include sexual assault, rape, sodomy, unwelcome touching, forced nudity, or taking unwanted naked pictures of the elderly person. Sexual abuse may involve physical violence, so many injury patterns of physical abuse may be seen. However, it is important to note some elders may have no physical evidence after sexual abuse, so the most important factor is the victim disclosing the event.

Signs and symptoms of sexual abuse:

- Bruises or injury to breast, buttocks, inner thighs, or anal/genital area
- Sexually transmitted infections
- Semen discovered in a female's urine

- Anogenital or urinary tract complaints (pain, dysuria, etc.) without etiology
- Fear or anxiety related to routine exam of genital area
- Torn or blood-stained undergarments
- Bleeding from anus or vagina

3. Neglect: Not providing for the elderly person's care or needs, such as food, hydration, shelter, hygiene, clothing, medical care, safety, and emotional and psychological well-being. The signs and symptoms of neglect may be seen in a variety of conditions and situations.

Signs and symptoms of neglect:

- Malnutrition and dehydration
- Malodorous body odor, unkempt appearance, inappropriate clothing or lack of clothing
- Untreated pressure ulcers, sores, or wounds
- Insect infestation
- Stool/urine smell
- Repeated missed medical appointments or delay of treatment
- Depression or anxiety

BOX 11.3 EXAMPLES OF REASONS FOR CAREGIVER ABUSE

- Caregiver burden, stress, advancing age, and handling his or her own medical issues
- Multiple role demands—adult child, parent, spouse, and so on
- Incompetent—does not understand the needs of the elder or is unaware of the available resources for support
- Financial burden
- Lack of support

4. Self-neglect: An older adult refuses or fails to provide for self and he or she engages in behavior that threatens his or her well-being, safety, and health, such as not consuming adequate food and water, not wearing appropriate clothes, insufficient hygiene, or not taking medications. Typically, elders who self-neglect have deficits in physical, cognitive, or functional abilities.

It is difficult to differentiate between neglect and self-neglect. If the patient is competent, simply asking if anyone is abusing him or her and having the elder disclose any information would be the most important factor.

Signs and symptoms of self-neglect:

- Homelessness, living in unsanitary places (dirt, bug infestation), or unsafe environments (no heat, faulty wires, no running water, fire hazards, etc.)
- Unkempt, dirty clothes or inappropriate clothes for the season
- Weight loss or dehydration
- Noncompliant with medicine or medical aids
- Does not keep medical appointments
- Refuses to leave his or her home

5. Emotional or psychological abuse: Verbally or nonverbally inflicting pain, anguish, or distress to the elder. This can include the "silent treatment," forced social isolation from friends or family, insults, humiliation, threats, harassment, intimidation, or belittling the elder in front of others.

   Signs and symptoms of emotional or psychological abuse:

- Depression, anxiety, noncommunication, agitated, or withdrawn
- Behavior that mimics dementia
- Self-soothing movement, such as rocking, talking to self, hugging self, sucking

6. Abandonment: The caregiver or the person who assumed the role of providing care to the elder deserted him or her.

   Signs and symptoms of abandonment:

- Elder deserted at a public place, such as a mall, park, bus station, or hospital

7. Financial and material exploitation: Using the elderly person's cash, property, or assets improperly or illegally. This includes forcing the elderly individual to sign over checks or the deeds to property by threatening to withhold care, forging his or her signature, taking cash from the elder, or stealing his or her possessions. Examples could be: a friend or family stating they will care for the elderly person for life if he or she signs over the property; a salesperson states the elderly person needs unnecessary repairs; someone provides false affection or coerces the elderly person to marry to defraud him or her of assets.

   Signs and symptoms of financial and material exploitation:

- Adding the caregiver's name to bank accounts or legal documents or large amounts of money being withdrawn
- Using the elder's automated teller machine (ATM) card without permission
- The elder's possessions or funds are disappearing
- Sudden changes in financial management

- The elder suddenly moves into someone else's house or has someone move into his or her house
- The elder is pushed quickly into making a financial transaction without being able to consult a trustworthy person
- Increase in checks being written out to "cash"
- The elder is being taken to different providers than he or she has been seeing in the past, such as lawyers, bankers, or healthcare providers

RED FLAG FINDINGS

- Unexplained injury or bruises
- The patient or caregiver has changed history multiple times
- History does not fit the elder's physical capabilities
- History does not explain or match the injury
- Delay in treatment
- Elder describes and reports the abuse

BOX 11.4 IMPACT OF ELDER ABUSE

- About 300% higher risk of death than those not abused
- Greater risk of hospitalization, emergency department (ED) visits, or placement in long-term-care facility
- Self-withdrawal, depression, anxiety, posttraumatic stress, and suicide ideation
- Decreased quality of life
- Digestive issues, chronic pain, hypertension, cardiac disease, and increased bone or joint problems
- Increased healthcare costs (Direct cost of injuries are estimated at more than $5.3 billion nationally; Chalise, 2017; Ho, Wong, Chiu, & Ho, 2017; Jett, 2016.)

SCREENING AND SCREENING TOOLS

The concept of screening comes from epidemiology, and the purpose of the screening tools is the early identification of the disease or disorder (in this case, elder abuse), so treatment can begin to decrease morbidity and mortality rates and increase quality of life (Leahy & Rosof-Williams, 2012; McCarthy, Campbell, & Penhale, 2017; Phelan & Treacy, 2011). Screening and screening tools for elder abuse are used to assist in the detection and identification of who is at risk of mistreatment or neglect, so the healthcare professional needs to have a sensitive, compassionate demeanor with thorough interviewing techniques. Screening tools should be reliable and valid and are evaluated by using statistical analysis of sensitivity and specificity; the perfect tool would have a high sensitivity and specificity value. Sensitivity helps to identify those who are being abused, which is referred to as a "true positive," and specificity helps identify those who are not being abused, which is a "true negative."

If the screening tool suggests potential abuse, further investigation and a more thorough interview process should be conducted with the elderly individual. It is vital to interview the elderly person alone. Some interview techniques involve active listening, guided questioning, nonverbal communication, empathetic responses, validation, and summarization. In addition to the interview techniques, setting the stage or framing direct questions about abuse is helpful in building a relationship and producing accurate information from the interviewees, which can include the victim, caregiver, and family member. Along with the screening process, healthcare providers must be able to identify cases that need to be reported to the authorities according to local state statutes.

BOX 11.5 EXAMPLE QUESTIONS FOR SETTING THE STAGE

Always ask all patients about violence in their lives because it is so common in our society. Have you or are you worried about violence or some form of abuse?

Unfortunately, people get taken advantage of financially and will receive phone calls, sometimes from family members, about bills or money owed. Do you have any concerns that this might be happening to you?

Sometimes elders do not get the help they need. Is this happening to you?

From past experience with other patients, I'm worried because these injuries or symptoms appear to be a result of abuse. Is someone hurting you?

Examples of Direct Questions

Do you feel safe where you live?

Is someone threatening you or hurting you (physically, emotionally, etc.)?

(continued)

BOX 11.5 EXAMPLE QUESTIONS FOR SETTING THE STAGE (*continued*)

Do you feel controlled or isolated?

Have you ever been hit, kicked, bitten, strangled, choked, slapped, pushed, or touched in any way that makes you uncomfortable?

Has anyone ever made you do anything sexual you did not want to?

Is someone withholding food, water, or shelter from you?

There are a number of well-known screening tools, but here is a list of a few.

The Elder Assessment Instrument (EAI): This tool takes about 15 minutes and is completed by a healthcare professional in a variety of clinical areas with a one-to-one interview and a physical assessment of the older adult. The tool encompasses both subjective and objective findings and is a 41-item scale subdivided into seven sections that relate to signs of abuse—general assessment, possible abuse, neglect, abandonment, exploitation indicators, and a summary section—but the tool does not assess psychological abuse. The revised version from 2012 is a 51-item adaptation from the previous scale and has captured financial and psychological abuse.

Elder Abuse Suspicion Index (EASI): Five questions are asked directly to the older adult that cover all aspects of abuse, and one observational question is for the provider to answer or is self-completed, thus eliminating any observational error. This tool is easy to use, takes less than 2 minutes, and is known to increase provider awareness. The tool was initially developed for physicians to use but has expanded to other healthcare professionals and settings. It is culturally transferable, has been translated into multiple languages, and is used in multiple countries.

The Hwalek–Sengstock Elder Abuse Screening Test (H-S EAST): This tool contains 15 items, but a 9-item version also exists that can be considered a direct questioning tool. It is a brief screening tool used best during the interview process and can be used in multiple settings. The tool screens for six different categories and includes a risk indicator for physical, neglect, material, emotional abuse, and a violation of personal rights.

The Older Adult Financial Exploitation Measure (OAFEM): This is the only validated financial screening tool. Adequate cognitive capacity is required, so a Mini-Mental Status Exam score of 17 or greater is needed for competency judgment by a healthcare professional. This is a 25-item tool that focuses on theft, scams, financial entitlement, coercion, money management, and symptoms of financial exploitation.

Brief Abuse Screen for the Elderly (BASE): This tool contains five questions, takes 1 minute to complete, and focuses on suspicion levels and abuse types. The use of the tool is limited and usually administered in conjunction with the Indicators of Abuse screening tool.

Indicators of Abuse (IOA): This tool is used to identify risk factors, not actual signs and symptoms. It has 27 indicator items used by a healthcare professional during an interview and usually in the home setting. The tool is easy to use because the items reflect a routine clinical exam, but this can result in clinical subjectivity. An expanded IOA has been developed to help with the subjectivity identified in the original IOA.

Screening for elder mistreatment varies and is limited for many reasons: There are no standards on how healthcare professionals should ask the elderly about abuse; there are varying abuse definitions; no universal screening tool exists; and there is unclear guidance about who should be screened and what to do if abuse is identified. The U.S. Preventive Services Task Force (USPSTF, 2013) concluded that the current evidence on the benefits and harms of screening all elderly adults is insufficient, although The Joint Commission requires accredited institutions to screen for violence and multiple professional organizations support the screening. Along with the screening process, healthcare providers must be able to identify cases that need to be reported to the authorities by local state statute and be vigilant of their state laws on reporting elder abuse.

Fast Facts

Healthcare professionals need to screen or ask about violence or abuse during every interaction with an elderly individual. Older adults are a vulnerable population and are at a higher risk for any form of abuse.

REPORTING ELDER ABUSE

Licensed nurses are mandatory reporters, and reporting suspected elder abuse is mandated in all 50 U.S. states and the District of Columbia (Jett, 2016; Leahy & Rosof-Williams, 2012; National Guideline Clearinghouse, 2013). A mandatory reporter is a person who is required to report any suspicion of abuse to the local authorities and the state, usually to a group called Adult Protective Services (APS). The purpose of APS is to protect and serve adults with disabilities and older adults who are being abused or are at risk of being abused. Each state developed an APS program because of the varying definitions of elder abuse, the states' elder population needs, and the states' resources. The American Bar Association provides an annual summary of state laws relating to elder abuse.

The reports are usually anonymous, but if the mandatory reporter feels the older adult is in immediate danger, the local authorities should be notified. The reporting varies based on the work setting. Every place of employment may be different, so know your institution's policies, but hospitals and nursing homes usually report internally first to the social worker and the social worker will then contact APS and/or local authorities. For home care settings, it is usually the nursing supervisor. Nursing homes and assisted-living facilities have an additional resource of contacting the state long-term-care ombudsman for help. If the nurse is a neighbor, friend, relative, or privately paid caregiver, he or she may be under obligation to report the abuse directly to APS. Every report to the ombudsman and to APS will be investigated.

Reporting elder mistreatment is different than child abuse because even if the elder is physically frail, but mentally competent, the older adult can refuse interventions. This means the elder cannot be removed from the harmful situation without his or her permission, which can be frustrating for healthcare professionals. Many states require reporting of specific injuries, such as ones caused by weapons as a result of violence or accidental mechanism, so if an elder patient seeks treatment with one of these injuries, a report is a requirement. Healthcare providers should inform elders if a report is necessary, educate them about the process, and answer any questions they may have.

If an older adult does not want to report his or her abuse, the healthcare provider should explore and address his or her concerns by explaining the benefits of reporting the abuse. It is important to provide further education to the elderly person about the process and continue to provide support and resources as needed.

Reporting and the Health Insurance Portability and Accountability Act (HIPAA) have caused some concerns and confusion over what information can be released to the investigators when the elderly individual did not sign a consent form or the nurse provided a mandated report. The HIPAA legislation permits hospitals, clinics, and the like to share protected information without the patient's consent when the covered entity reasonably believes the patient is a victim. Plus, if abuse is considered, the U.S. Department of Health and Human Services allows hospitals, clinics, and the like to share the protected health information with local and state authorities. Again, healthcare professionals need to understand their own workplace policies related to reporting and the local state laws about abuse and privacy issues.

CONCLUSION

Elder maltreatment is a serious issue in society and rates of elder abuse will increase as the general population ages and lives longer; so too will this population be at risk for elder maltreatment. Forensic nurses and nurses who work with elders are in a key position to screen, identify, and provide linkage and resources to those most vulnerable and at risk. It is imperative that nurses have a foundational knowledge in elder maltreatment so that they can help patients who may be experiencing any types of abuse and address this serious public health problem.

RESOURCES

National Center on Elder Abuse (NCEA)—(855) 500-3537, https://ncea.acl. gov/resources/state.html. This website offers direct links to state information, whom to contact and their phone numbers, other helplines, and referral sources.

Eldercare Locator—(800) 677-1116, https://eldercare.acl.gov/Public/Index. aspx. It is sponsored by the U.S. Administration on Aging and refers you to the appropriate agency in your area to report the suspected abuse.

Adult Protective Services—(202) 370-6292, www.napsa-now.org/get-help/ help-in-your-area. Each state has an APS program and the website offers direct state information.

National Long-Term-Care Ombudsman Program—(202) 332-2275, theconsumervoice.org/get_help. Each state has a long-term-care ombudsman program and the website offers direct state information.

National Association of Area Agencies on Aging—(202) 872-0888, https:// www.n4a.org. This website offers information on all resources available in your community.

ConsultGeri.org, https://consultgeri.org. This website is an evidence-based geriatric clinical nursing website that offers webinars and assessment tools for elder mistreatment.

References

Chalise, H. N. (2017). Elder abuse: A neglected issue in developing countries. *Jacobs Journal of Gerontology*, 3(1), 24.

Emergency Nurses Association. (2014). Surface and burn trauma. In D. Gurney (Ed.), *Trauma nursing core course* (7th ed., pp. 205–224). Des Plaines, IL: Emergency Nurses Association.

Eisikovits, Z., Winterstein, T., & Lowenstein, A. (2004). The national survey on elder abuse and neglect in Israel. Retrieved from http://www.inpea.net/images/Israel_NationalSurvey2004.pdf

Faircloth, E. (2016). Elder abuse: Our responsibilities in society and in healthcare. *Synergy: Imaging & Therapy Practice*, August 1, pp. 5–10. Retrieved from https://www.sor.org/system/files/article/201606/io_2016_lr.pdf#page=10

Ho, C. H., Wong, S. Y., Chiu, M. M., & Ho, R. M. (2017). Global prevalence of elder abuse: A meta-analysis and meta-regression. *East Asian Archives of Psychiatry, 27*(2), 43–55.

Jett, K. (2016). Common legal and ethical issues. In T. A. Touhy & K. Jett (Eds.), *Ebersole & Hess' toward healthy aging human needs and nursing response* (9th ed., pp. 417–426). St. Louis, MO: Elsevier.

Leahy, L. G., & Rosof-Williams, J. (2012). Psychosocial health problems. In J. G. Whetstone Foster & S. S. Prevost (Eds.), *Advanced practice nursing of adults in acute care* (pp. 98–174). Philadelphia, PA: F.A. Davis.

Maryland Department of Health. (2008). Patterned bruises. Retrieved from https://phpa.health.maryland.gov/mch/Documents/MDChamp/CHAMP-Handbook-2008-Patterned-Bruising.pdf

McCarthy, L., Campbell, S., & Penhale, B. (2017). Elder abuse screening tools: A systematic review. *The Journal of Adult Protection, 19*(6), 368–379. doi:10.1108/JAP-10-2016-0026

National Guideline Clearinghouse. (2013). Guideline summary: Screening for intimate partner violence and abuse of elderly and vulnerable adults: U.S. Preventive Services Task Force recommendation statement. Retrieved from https://www.guideline.gov/summaries/summary/39425/screening-for-intimate-partner-violence-and-abuse-of-elderly-and-vulnerable-adults-us-preventive-services-task-force-recommendation-statement?q=elder+abuse

Phelan, A., & Treacy, M. P. (2011). *A review of elder abuse screening tools, NCPOP, School of Nursing,* Midwifery and Health Systems, University College Dublin. Retrieved from http://www.ncpop.ie/userfiles/file/ncpop%20reports/538_NCPOP-proof7.pdf

Pillemer, K., Burnes, D., Riffin, C., & Lachs, M. S. (2016). Elder abuse: Global situation, risk factors, and prevention strategies. *Gerontologist, 56*, S194–S205. doi:10.1093/geront/gnw004

Tully, J. (2015). Bruising—Can we really tell which bruises are caused by abuse? Retrieved from https://www.rch.org.au/uploadedFiles/Main/Content/vfpms/7_VFPMS%20seminar2015%20Bruising%20RCH%20format_ni.pdf

World Health Organization (WHO). (2018). Elder abuse: Fact sheet. Retrieved from http://www.who.int/mediacentre/factsheets/fs357/en

12

Bullying

Meredith J. Scannell

Bullying is an everlasting problem that impacts the well-being as well as the academic and financial health of those affected. Bullying is a form of violence associated with school-aged children; however it can occur among adults and in the work setting. Forensic nurses have the educational background and experience to identify those at risk and those in current situations and can be champions in addressing the issue and bringing it to the forefront. They bring awareness to this everlasting problem and the impact it has on those it affects.

At the end of the chapter, the nurse will be able to:

1. Describe the different types of bullying and those most vulnerable.
2. Understand the physical, mental, academic, and financial impact of the various types of bullying.
3. List strategies in addressing bullying and engaging other professionals in addressing the problem.

BACKGROUND

Bullying is the repeated harmful acts of physical or psychological intimidation over time directed toward an individual, creating an imbalance of physical or psychological power. Forms of bullying can be direct or indirect. Direct bullying includes acts that are committed directly to the individual, such as physical assault and name-calling. Indirect bullying includes acts that are committed indirectly to the individual, such as spreading harmful rumor about the individual. Other forms of bullying can exist and may be financial, sexual, or even social. Bullying is widespread and a common experience for children and adolescents in schools across all grade levels. In 2015 a national study showed one in five high school students has reported being bullied on school grounds within the last year (CDC, 2016).

VICTIMS OF BULLYING

Victims of bullying often tend to be socially isolated, have low self-esteem, and are unlikely to defend themselves or retaliate. They often are much weaker and smaller than their peers and nonassertive, often exhibiting lower levels of self esteem and lower social skills (Matthiesen & Einarsen, 2015).

Characteristics of victims of bullying include the following:

- Younger age
- Low self-esteem
- Ethnic, cultural, or religious minority
- Poor social skills
- LGBTQI individuals
- Obesity
- Health or medical conditions
- Learning disabilities
- Physical disabilities

Fast Facts

Although bullying often relates to children, adults can also experience different types of bullying

Effects of bullying can have a significant negative impact on the victim and can lead to long- and short-term health consequences (Jones, Waite & Clements, 2012). Mental health effects of bullying can lead to anxiety, depression, and self-harm. Somatic symptoms of bullying include stomachaches, sleeping disorders, headaches, dizziness, and back pain. Physical injuries can include wounds, broken bones, burns, and poisoning (Peyton, Ranasinghe, & Jacobsen, 2017). One serious health consequence is suicide. A large body of research has demonstrated a strong link between bullying and suicide. A large meta-analysis study conducted by Moore et al. (2017) demonstrated a fourfold increase in suicide attempts among individuals who were frequently bullied. There is also a reproductive health effect among some victims of bullying, such as teenage pregnancy, risky sexual behavior, and early-onset sexual behavior. Bullying also can have a negative effect on maladaptive behaviors in the victim and lead to recreational drug and alcohol misuse. Bullying can also have an impact on the academic performance of the individual and his or her ability to participate fully in academic programs. The school environment becomes hostile for the student and can impact the level of concentration and desire to engage in school activities, and it may lead to low grades and frequent absenteeism in attempts to avoid bullying.

TYPES OF BULLYING

There are many different forms of bullying; discussed here are the most common types of bullying. Table 12.1 provides an overview of the different types of bullying.

Physical Bullying

Physical bullying includes the direct physical acts that are done to cause fear and intimidation over the individual. It entails hitting, pinching, punching, or pulling hair. It can also be less obvious, such as tripping the individual, making it look like it was the victim's clumsiness. Other physical acts can be the destruction of the individual's property, such as books, notebooks, and phones. In some cases, the physical acts can be extreme, such as hazing.

Verbal Bullying

Verbal bullying comprises nonphysical acts that impact the psyche of the individual. Intimidation is one form of psychological bullying that is often harder to notice. It is an intentional action that seriously threatens and induces a sense of fear or inferiority upon the victim. Verbal acts that have a direct impact include name-calling or teasing.

Sexual Bullying

Sexual bullying is a common type of bullying and includes acts of a sexual nature in which sexuality or gender is used against the individual. These acts can be different forms of physical contact and fall under sexual assault and sexual violence. Sexual bullying can also be verbal and includes sexual harassment with sexual comments

Table 12.1

Example of Types of Bullying

Type of Bullying	Examples
Physical	■ Physical assaults and injuries to the individual: hitting, punching, pinching, or pushing ■ Attacking with a weapon ■ Tripping ■ Hazing ■ Something thrown at the individual ■ Damaging property ■ Destroying work, physically breaking something, or writing on it ■ Theft of possessions
Verbal	■ Intimidation ■ Name-calling ■ Comments about race, nationality, or religion ■ Comments about body parts or looks ■ Threats to an individual or the individuals's property ■ Demands for money or other goods
Sexual	■ Sexual assault ■ Touching of body parts ■ Sexual harassment ■ Having to wear provocative clothing ■ Comments about gender or sexuality ■ Making sexual gestures ■ Attempting to take off the individual's clothing
Social	■ Malicious gossiping or spreading rumors ■ Ignoring, excluding or ostracizing from activities or other people for various reasons ■ Being locked inside ■ Attempts to turn others against the person
Cyber	■ Sending threatening or harmful emails ■ Posting threats or messages that are harmful on personal or the victim's social media ■ Posting or sharing humiliating or personal photos or fake photos of the individual without permission ■ Taking pictures or videos of the person without his or her permission for the purpose of humiliating or harming
Work	■ Constant and unfair criticism ■ Yelling, shouting, and screaming ■ Insults and behind-the-back put-downs ■ Monopolizing supplies and other resources ■ Aggressive emails or notes ■ Sending emails at unreasonable times and expecting immediate response

to the individual. It can also include rumors and gossip that contain sexual aspects, such as someone being sexually active and what he or she did. Research has also shown individuals of the LGBT community experience higher rates of sexually bullying, in which acts regarding their sexual identity and gender are used in efforts to humiliate or degrade the individual. Cyber aspects of sexual bullying include sending sexual photos or messages to the individual or sharing pictures of a sexual nature of the person to others without his or her consent. Other forms of sexual bullying may include acts in which someone else is forced or pressured to perform acts of sexual assault on another person in to conduct on another person.

Social Bullying

Social bullying more often includes covert types of bullying and is harder to identify. Social bullying entails acts of ignoring the individual or ostracizing the person from activities and other groups, thereby limiting interactions with others. It also includes acts such as gossiping about the individual and spreading rumors, which can have a direct impact on the individual.

Cyberbullying constitutes acts of harassing, humiliating, intimidating, or threatening others over the Internet or other methods of technology. Unlike other types of bullying, cyberbullies may know their victim and are able to remain anonymous. Cyberbullying can also have a much broader impact, as information is shared over electronic devices to large audiences, and it can occur at any time of the day, unlike school-based bullying, which occurs only during school time. The impact of cyberbullying can be greater as it is harder to take down or stop a cyberbully.

Workplace bullying is the deliberate, repeated mistreatment of individuals within the work setting. It can include intentional humiliation, intimidation, and sabotage of performance. Bullying in the work setting can occur at and between any levels within the organization, such as bullying between coworkers and bullying between a supervisor and subordinate. Forms of bullying in the workplace can be direct acts, such as threatening employees, or less obvious acts, such as creating unreasonable deadlines for work assignments.

Fast Facts

Bullying can take on different forms and often people will experience more than one individual type of bullying.

BULLIES

Children, adolescents, and young adults who bully often like to feel in control. They are narcissistic and have little empathy for the victims, and acts they commit result in their own personal satisfaction. They defend, justify, or blame the victim for their actions. They exhibit higher levels of aggression compared to those who don't bully (Matthiesen & Einarsen, 2015). Bullies also engage in other high risk and maladaptive behaviors, such as drinking alcohol and recreational drug use and engaging in other criminal activities such as stealing and property destruction. In addition, children and young adults who bully often become adults who bully.

Males bully more often than females and will bully both males and females, whereas females who bully are most likely to bully other females. Bullies usually do not engage in their activities alone and typically have other peers involved. Some peers may join in and assist the bully and others may support the bully by providing an audience, laughing, taunting, or encouraging the bullying.

ASSESSING FOR BULLYING

Bullying is often underreported, as the victim may fear retaliation, feel shameful for not standing up for self, fear of not being believed, or fear that the problem will become worse if the bullying is reported (Milnes, et al., 2015). Educational efforts should address how students and others can report bullying without putting themselves in further risk or harm (Milnes, et al., 2015). Other educational efforts should address how healthcare professionals and others can directly assess for bullying or assess for red flags that may indicate bullying. Protective measures against bullying include a school climate that promotes safety, respect, and kindness to others (Milnes, et al., 2015). Antibully programs are more effective in young children and efforts should be made to prioritize education at an early age. Healthcare professionals working with school-aged individuals should assess for bullying and have a uniform approach for dealing with it.

STRATEGIES TO PREVENT BULLYING

- Educate parents and teachers about bullying
- Whole school training and education
- Parental support
- Playground supervision
- Classroom management and rules

- Universal policies against bullying
- Disciplinary methods for bullying

CONCLUSION

Bullying is a serious public health problem that can lead to adverse health outcomes. Bullying is modifiable and preventable and should be addressed at multiple levels and not solely in the school system. Nurses who work with school-aged individuals are in a key position to screen for bullying and monitor for its signs and symptoms, helping to combat this significant public health problem.

RESOURCES

National Parent Information Network: www.npin.org
Educators for Social Responsibility: www.benjerry.com/esr/about~esr.html
Bullying in Schools and What to Do About It: www.education.unisa.edu.au/ bullying
Anti-Bullying Network: www.antibullying.net
National Youth Violence Prevention Resource Center: www.safeyouth.org/ scripts/topics/school.asp
Federal Bureau of Investigation—Resources on School Violence: www.fbi. gov/page2/april07/addtnresources.htm
Keep Schools Safe—School Safety, Security and Violence Prevention Resources: www.keepschoolssafe.org
PTA Organization—School Violence: www.pta.org/topicschoolviolence.asp
Consortium to Prevent School Violence: www.preventschoolviolence.org

References

Centers for Disease Control and Prevention (CDC). (2016). Youth risk behavior surveillance—United States, 2015. *Morbidity and Mortality Weekly Report, Surveillance Summaries, 65*(SS9). Retrieved from http://www.cdc. gov/mmwr/volumes/65/ss/ss6506a1.htm.

Jones, S. N., Waite, R., & Thomas Clements, P. (2012). An evolutionary concept analysis of school violence: From bullying to death. *Journal of Forensic Nursing, 8*(1), 4–12. doi:10.1111/j.1939-3938.2011.01121.x

Matthiesen, S. B., & Einarsen, S. (2015). Perpetrators and targets of bullying at work: Role stress and individual differences. In *Perspectives on bullying: Research on childhood, workplace, and cyberbullying* (pp. 135–154). New York, NY: Springer Publishing.

Milnes, K., Turner-Moore, T., Gough, B., Denison, J., Gatere, L., Haslam, C., . . . Zoppi, I. (2015). Sexual bullying in young people across five European countries: Research report for the Addressing Sexual Bullying Across Europe (ASBAE) Project. Retrieved from http://webcache. googleusercontent.com/search?q=cache:DxkLKvROBMwJ:ec.europa.eu/ justice/grants/results/daphne-toolkit/en/file/2924/download%3Ftoken% 3DLR_7bJf5+&cd=1&hl=en&ct=clnk&gl=in

Moore, S. E., Norman, R. E., Suetani, S., Thomas, H. J., Sly, P. D., & Scott, J. G. (2017). Consequences of bullying victimization in childhood and adolescence: A systematic review and meta-analysis. *World Journal of Psychiatry, 7*(1), 60–76. doi:10.5498/wjp.v7.i1.60

Peyton, R. P., Ranasinghe, S., & Jacobsen, K. H. (2017). Injuries, violence, and bullying among middle school students in Oman. *Oman Medical Journal, 32*(2), 98–105. doi:10.5001/omj.2017.19

IV

Community and Global Violence

13

Community Violence

Meredith J. Scannell

Community violence is a public health problem of epidemic proportions with devastating effects on the health and well-being of many patients. Community-related violence includes acts of violence that occur outside of the family and relationships and involves youth violence, acquaintance and stranger violence, violence related to property crimes, and violence in workplaces and other institutions. Community violence refers to the intentional use of physical force or power, threatened or actual, against another person or against a group within the community. The effects of the violence can lead to injury, death, psychological harm, maldevelopment, or deprivation. It is essential for providers to understand the overlapping experiences of traumatic events for patients while providing the highest quality of care.

At the end of the chapter, the nurse will be able to:

1. Describe the different types of community violence and the impact they have on individuals, families, and communities.
2. Identify actual signs and red flags of individuals associated with or at risk for gang activities or involvement.
3. List strategies to improve workplace violence.

BACKGROUND

Community violence is a serious public health problem that impacts the lives and well-being of individuals, families, neighborhoods, and communities. Those disproportionately affected by violence include those who live in low-income and underserved populations. Growing up in areas of violence can impact stress levels, perceptions of what is normal, and health. Constant exposure to violence can lead to social isolation, a feeling of being unsafe, anxiety, and depression. It is essential for nurses in all settings to identify those at risk and address the issue so that the health and lives of people are not impacted. In 2016, 15.9 million property crimes occurred in the United States, which includes burglary and theft, and 9% of households experienced at least one type of property damage.

HATE CRIME

Hate crimes are crimes that occur with a motivation against an individual's race, sexual orientation, or gender; religious background; disability; or national group. Hate crimes may include direct assaults, sexual assaults, degradation or attacking of personal property or places of worship, harassment, and vandalism. Hate crimes occur more often when there are poor or uncertain economic conditions.

GANG VIOLENCE

Gang violence is a serious problem affecting numerous individuals and communities. Gangs are groups of people of at least three to six individuals who engage in a pattern of criminal activity and often have a hierarchy, alliance or understanding, and identities by a common name, symbol, or sign (Akiyama, 2012). Gang members individually or collectively engage in an ongoing pattern of criminal or delinquent activity. Belonging to a gang is strongly linked to criminal activity, such as homicides, burglaries, and selling of illicit substances. Gangs may be motivated by money, and they may not be committed to a specific neighborhood but move from location to location; gangs are motivated by claiming a "turf" or neighborhood in which they do their criminal activity (Akiyama, 2012).

Individuals join gangs for various reasons. Some people seek fun and excitement and gangs can be attractive to younger individuals who watch news and media. And the music industry glamorizes the gang lifestyle. Other people join gangs for a sense of identity and belonging, as they can represent ties, through racial or ethnic backgrounds, and give a sense of family to those who lack a stable home life or family.

Peer pressure can also be an influence on some to join a gang. They join without an understanding of what a gang is and the risks associated with it. Family tradition may also dictate joining a gang as a second- and third-generation gang member, because an older brother or sister is a gang member. Lastly, joining can offer a sense of protection, especially for individuals who are in an environment and community in which there is danger, such as prisons and gang-affiliated neighborhoods; joining a gang guarantees support in cases of assault.

Fast Facts

Hand signs are used to show allegiance to a specific gang.

INDICATORS OF GANG ASSOCIATION

Openly admitting to being involved in a gang

Changing appearance with specific haircut or clothing piece, such as a bandana of a certain color

Wearing clothing in a certain way, such as one pant leg rolled up

Wearing a jewel with a specific design or symbol, or worn in a specific way

Requesting a specific brand of clothing

New markings such as a tattoo or symbol

Using hand signs

Graffiti on personal items or having graffiti paraphernalia

Change in behavior toward those in authority or family

Carrying weapons

Disobeying rules

Changing friends

Having a sudden increase in money or possessions

WORKPLACE VIOLENCE

Workplace violence is a worldwide serious health and occupational hazard to some individuals and in some professions. In 2016 the U.S.

Bureau of Labor Statistics reported 500 homicides in the work setting out of a total of 5,190 fatal work injuries in the United States. Actual numbers of nonfatal workplace violence are difficult to determine, as the numbers for intentional and nonintentional violence injuries are not collected and many other acts of violence may not involve injuries (Bureau of Labor Statistics, 2018). Workplace violence tends to occur more often in industries such as law enforcement, healthcare, and the military. It has been reported that one-third of all nurses have experienced some kind of workplace violence. Nurses in all settings are at risk with some of the highest risks occurring in psychiatry, geriatrics, emergency departments (EDs), and correctional facilities (Spector, Zhou, & Che, 2014). There are several different types of violence, including physical contact most often made by patients but also by family members, other visitors, and other members of the healthcare team (Spector, Zhou, & Che, 2014). Other types of workplace violence can include nonphysical violence, verbal violence, bullying, and sexual harassment.

RECOMMENDED STRATEGIES TO ADDRESS WORKPLACE VIOLENCE

- Educate employees on work-related violence prevention and management policies and procedures.
- Define workplace violence with a distinction between unintentional assaults due to medication or mental health and intentional assaults due to drugs or alcohol.
- Encourage a zero-tolerance policy on workplace violence.
- Recognize early signs of escalation.
- Identify individual and environmental risk factors for violence.
- Conduct personal safety training.
- Advocate for local and state laws on healthcare personnel violence.

PREVENTION

Nurses play an important role in addressing the issue of community violence. Nurses work in all settings, including those where they are likely to come across individuals facing different forms of community violence, such as in schools, health centers, and EDs. Nurses can assess for high-risk factors. Community outreach or partnership with community violence prevention programs and refer individuals who are at high risk those at risk. Some communities have violence recovery specialists who work in conjunction with multidisciplinary teams to offer ongoing advocacy and resources to those at risk.

The Emergency Nurses Association (2018) has an online tool-kit that addresses workplace violence. It contains relevant research notes, assessment tools, and educational material.

CONCLUSION

Community violence is a serious problem that disproportionately affects those who live in low-income and underserved communities. Having an understanding of the different types of violence and those at risk can equip nurses to address the issue and provide linkage to necessary prevention services. Nurses in all healthcare settings have a responsibility to address this problem, which is essential for the lives and health of individuals, families, neighborhoods, and communities.

References

Akiyama, C. (2012). Understanding youth street gangs. *Journal of Emergency Nursing, 38*(6), 568–570. doi:10.1016/j.jen.2011.10.006

Bureau of Labor Statistics (BLS). (2018). *There were 500 workplace homicides in the United States in 2016.* United States Department of Labor. Retrieved from https://www.bls.gov/opub/ted/2018/there-were-500-workplace-homicides -in-the-united-states-in-2016.htm?view_full

Emergency Nurses Association. (2018). Workplace violence toolkit. Retrieved from https://www.ena.org/docs/default-source/resource-libr ary/practice-resources/toolkits/workplaceviolencetoolkit.pdf?sfvrsn =6785bc04_28

Spector, P. E., Zhou, Z. E., & Che, X. X. (2014). Nurse exposure to physical and nonphysical violence, bullying, and sexual harassment: A quantitative review. *International Journal of Nursing Studies, 51*(1), 72–84. doi:10.1016/j.ijnurstu.2013.01.010

14

Strangulation

Andrea MacDonald

Strangulation can be an undetected risk factor for victims of intimate partner violence (IPV) that exponentially increases risk for lethal injury. "Strangulation" is defined as the reduction of blood flow and oxygenation to or from the brain that occurs from external compression of the blood vessels in the neck. Strangulation can be accomplished via multiple methods and can be difficult to detect. Strangulation is a red flag that indicates escalation of IPV and increases risk of lethality. The World Health Organization (WHO) states that women are six times more likely than men to experience strangulation as a form of IPV. The lethality risk for strangulation victims is of critical significance. History of prior nonfatal strangulation has been associated with more than six times greater likelihood of progression to attempted homicide and more than seven times greater likelihood of progression to completed homicide.

Strangulation may not leave visible physical signs. Symptoms experienced poststrangulation may mimic other medical issues and therefore go unidentified as sequelae of strangulation. Although some victims of strangulation may be identified during episodic care, it is more likely that victims will not disclose IPV. The inability of victims of IPV to disclose often chronic/frequent histories of physical assault, including strangulation, creates a challenge for forensic nurses to accurately assess, detect, and treat victims of IPV who experience strangulation. This chapter describes the signs and symptoms of strangulation, gives information on screening and treatment of victims during episodic care, and provides guidance for assisting victims toward aftercare resources.

At the end of the chapter, the nurse will be able to:

- Define strangulation and understand the high risk that strangulation poses to lethality for victims of IPV.
- Identify populations that may be at risk for strangulation.
- Understand the signs and symptoms of strangulation.
- Differentiate between strangulation and choking and assist victims to differentiate.
- Identify resources for victims of IPV and strangulation.

BACKGROUND

Nonfatal strangulation has been identified as a high risk for homicide (particularly for women) for decades. The National Mortality Followback Survey (NMFS) in 1993 indicated that the risk for women dying from strangulation was approximately 10% higher than for men and that 68% of women reporting IPV also reported strangulation by their abusers. Strangulation was cited as the cause of lethal injury in IPV with approximately 5% more frequency than other methods of abuser violence (Funk & Schuppel, 2003). Strangulation accounts for 10% of all homicides in the United States (Glass et al., 2008). While this is statistically significant, an equally troubling issue is that most strangulation victims survive and may experience significant health issues poststrangulation that impair the ability of the victim to live a productive life. Increased risk of death is paramount for survivors of strangulation. Absence of external findings often leaves victims of strangulation untreated or undertreated. Undetected strangulation increases risk of lethality for victims. Accurate strangulation assessment by nurses is essential to the survival and wellness of victims of IPV.

TYPES OF STRANGULATION

- *Hanging:* use of a ligature (cord-like object such as rope or clothing) to suspend victim above ground that results in obstruction of blood/oxygen flow between lungs, heart, and brain/

compression of trachea/injury of cervical spinal cord, causing temporary/permanent injury or death.

- **Manual:** use of bare hands to compress neck area that results in obstruction of blood/oxygen flow between lungs, heart, and brain/compression of trachea/injury of cervical spinal cord, causing temporary/permanent injury or death. Manual strangulation is the most common form of strangulation in IPV.

  Manual strangulation is also known as "throttling" or "choking/choking out."

- **Chokehold:** use of a body part, usually a forearm, applied by the assailant from behind the victim to compress neck area that results in obstruction of blood/oxygen flow between lungs, heart, and brain/compression of trachea/injury of cervical spinal cord, causing temporary/permanent injury or death. The chokehold can also be performed with the victim lying prone and the assailant placing a knee, extremity, or an object across the neck of the victim and applying force.

  Chokehold strangulation is also known as "postural strangulation."

- **Ligature:** use of a cord-like object such as a rope, a belt, an article of clothing or an electrical cord to compress neck area that results in obstruction of blood/oxygen flow between lungs, heart, and brain/compression of trachea/injury of cervical spinal cord, causing temporary/permanent injury or death.

  Ligature strangulation is also known as "garroting."

It is important to use terminology that victims understand when performing a strangulation assessment. Many victims do not recognize that strangulation and choking indicate different mechanisms. During a strangulation assessment, the nurse may use the terms "strangle" and "choke" interchangeably to insure victims fully understand what is being asked of them. During documentation, the term "strangulation" should always be used to indicate the nature of assault.

AT-RISK POPULATIONS

Any person can be at risk for strangulation. High-risk populations include women of all ages but especially younger and socioeconomically disenfranchised, disabled, and cohabitating women (Sorenson, Joshi, & Sivitx, 2014). African American women were noted to have a slightly higher occurrence of strangulation than Latina women, Caucasian women, or other racial/ethnic groups but were less likely to experience fatal strangulation. In a study of female strangulation victims in San Diego, nearly 90% of strangulation victims had a previous history of IPV and more than 80% of these victims had physical and/or psychiatric symptoms related to being strangled. Strangulation is more commonly seen in heterosexual partners but may be underreported in same-sex couples as many studies have excluded same-sex partners. Individuals involved in marriages, cohabitating, and dating have been documented as having the greatest degree of strangulation as a form of IPV. IPV can, however, extend beyond the demise of an intimate partner relationship and may even occur when an intimate relationship has never existed. Strangulation by ex-partners and stalkers does occur (Pritchard, Reckdenwald, & Nordham, 2017). The U.S. Preventative Task Force recommends that all women between the ages of 14 and 46 be screened for IPV risk (United States Preventative Task Force, 2013). It is essential that the nurse do a thorough social assessment when screening for possible strangulation/IPV.

THE STRANGULATION ASSESSMENT

Assessment for strangulation can be challenging as there are often no obvious signs and/or symptoms. Victims may not report, may minimize events, or may not recall being strangled due to the use of substance or due to direct results of strangulation that can impair memory. As previously noted, terminology used by nursing staff may not be familiar to victims and result in failure to report. Fear of the perpetrator may also lead to nonreporting by victims. Screening questions must be asked in a sensitive and patient-centered manner.

Nurses can use best practice and clinical judgment to create a dialogue that is patient-focused and easily understood by patients so that clear and effective communication between nurse and patient occurs. Effective questions that can lead to disclosure are:

- Have you ever been strangled or choked by anyone?
- What was used to strangle/choke you?
- How long did the strangling/choking last?
- Were you shaken by the person who strangled/choked you?
- How many times were you strangled/choked?
- Did you pass out/lose consciousness when you were strangled/choked?

These questions can be tailored to the age/intellectual level/culture of the victims by changing the wording as necessary.

In addition to questioning, clinical observation must be part of the strangulation assessment. Victims may not realize that symptoms they are experiencing are related to strangulation. The skilled forensic nurse must align signs and symptoms to the narrative that a patient offers and also consider the emotional/physical cues that a patient may offer during the assessment. Suspicion for IPV/strangulation should occur when the patient story does not seem consistent with the presentation for care or when the patient has a documented history of IPV/strangulation. Well-developed communication skills must be paired with clinical assessment skills for accurate evaluation and care of strangulation victims.

SIGNS AND SYMPTOMS OF STRANGULATION

Strangulation can be insidious as it often leaves no physical signs or symptoms and victims may not report strangulation when presenting for care. When strangulation is reported or suspected, a comprehensive medical evaluation should occur.

Table 14.1 provides a review of systems along with the signs and symptoms of strangulation and focused nursing assessments/interventions.

Table 14.1

Signs and Symptoms of Strangulation and Nursing Assessments/Interventions		
System	Signs and Symptoms	Assessments/Interventions
■ Neurological	■ Headache ■ Altered mental status ■ Cerebrovascular accident ■ Anoxic brain injury ■ Loss of memory/ consciousness ■ Seizures ■ Learning deficit ■ Incontinence	■ Glasgow Coma Scale ■ Cranial nerve assessment ■ Motor function assessment ■ Pupillary response ■ CT scan of head/neck ■ MRI head/neck ■ Analgesia ■ Symptomatic treatment
■ Cardiovascular	■ Cardiac arrhythmias ■ Carotid artery dissection ■ Vasovagal syncope ■ Cardiac arrest	■ ECG ■ Cardiac telemetry ■ Echocardiogram ■ Cardiac testing ■ CPR/ACLS ■ Analgesia ■ Symptomatic treatment

(continued)

Table 14.1

Signs and Symptoms of Strangulation and Nursing Assessments/Interventions (*continued*)

System	Signs and Symptoms	Assessments/Interventions
■ Eyes	■ Periorbital petechiae ■ Subconjunctival hemorrhage ■ Vision changes	■ Visual acuity ■ Ocular pressure measurement ■ Evaluation of retinal arteries ■ Ophthalmology consultation ■ Analgesia ■ Symptomatic treatment
■ Ears	■ Bruising behind ears ■ Tinnitus	■ Hearing evaluation ■ Skin assessment ■ Analgesia ■ Symptomatic treatment
■ Mouth	■ Swelling/edema of the lips/tongue/uvula ■ Petechial hemorrhage of the tongue, gingiva, or oral palate	■ Oral assessment ■ Analgesia ■ Symptomatic treatment
■ Neck/Throat	■ Injury to the skin ■ Sore throat ■ Difficulty/pain with swallowing ■ Vocal distortion ■ Hyoid bone injury/fracture ■ Esophageal trauma/edema	■ Speech/swallow assessment ■ Radiology studies ■ CT scan ■ Infection prophylaxis ■ Forensic evidence collection ■ Analgesia ■ Symptomatic treatment
■ Respiratory	■ Changes in breathing patterns ■ Pulmonary edema ■ Aspiration/aspiration pneumonia ■ Respiratory distress	■ Respiratory assessment ■ Chest x-ray ■ CT scan ■ Infection prophylaxis ■ Analgesia ■ Symptomatic treatment
■ Reproductive	■ Spontaneous abortion ■ Sexually transmitted infection ■ Irregular or heavy menses ■ Unwanted pregnancies	■ Gynecological assessment ■ Pelvic examination ■ Pelvic ultrasound ■ Laboratory tests ■ Analgesia ■ Symptomatic treatment

(*continued*)

Table 14.1

System	Signs and Symptoms	Assessments/Interventions
■ Psychiatric	■ Behavioral changes ■ Anxiety/depression ■ PTSD ■ Insomnia ■ Suicidal/homicidal Ideation ■ Hypervigilance/paranoia ■ Personality changes	■ Psychiatric assessment ■ Suicidality/homicidality screening ■ Supportive therapies ■ Safety measures ■ Aftercare ■ Analgesia ■ Symptomatic treatment
■ Musculoskeletal	■ Bone fractures ■ Tendon/ligament/muscle injuries	■ Radiology studies ■ Supportive therapies ■ Analgesia ■ Symptomatic treatment
■ Integumentary	■ Trauma to skin such as laceration, abrasion, bruising, ligature marks, or pattern injury (finger marks) ■ Defensive wounds to hand/arms/legs ■ Injuries to face, neck, chest, scalp, and postauricular areas	■ Skin assessment ■ Wound care ■ Infection prophylaxis ■ Forensic evidence collection (including photography) ■ Analgesia ■ Symptomatic treatment

ACLS, advanced cardiovascular life support; CPR, cardiopulmonary resuscitation; PTSD, posttraumatic stress disorder.
Source: Adapted from Scannell, M., MacDonald, A. E., & Foster, C. (2017). Strangulation: What every nurse must recognize. *Nursing Made Incredibly Easy, 15,* 41–46. doi:10.1097/01.NME.00005255552.06539.02

IMPLICATIONS FOR FORENSIC NURSES

Detection of strangulation injuries can literally be the difference between life and death for victims of IPV. Nonlethal strangulation has significant and often long-term negative consequences that affect not only the health of the victim but the ability of the victim to engage in a meaningful and positive manner within the greater society. Nonlethal strangulation also presents an extreme risk for progression to lethality. Victims who survive strangulation can also experience physical and mental sequelae that result in a significant impact to both the individual and society. The social and financial consequences of IPV/strangulation cannot be tolerated and heavily damage humanity. Forensic nurses have a clinical and ethical mandate to identify strangulation as a crime so that policies and laws can support punishment for perpetrators and provide justice for victims.

Forensic nurses must assess and properly document strangulation so that proper clinical treatment can be implemented. Precise documentation is essential to legal proceedings that facilitate victim advocacy. The role of the forensic nurse is to treat victims of strangulation for physical, emotional, or psychiatric consequences as well as to collect valuable evidence of criminal malice so that victims can move toward the highest level of health restoration possible. Understanding the signs and symptoms of strangulation and essential treatment/documentation strategies is critical to ensure that victims receive the best care possible. Forensic evidence collection along with forensic photography is essential for proper documentation of all strangulation events. It is the duty of the forensic nurse to demonstrate knowledge and proficiency in caring for victims of strangulation.

Fast Facts

When documenting injuries, the patient may need to come back in a day or so, as some injuries take time to show marks, or having the patient return for future documentation can show different stages of healing.

CONCLUSION

Strangulation occurs in IPV and has an extremely high risk of lethality. Forensic nurses must understand both real-time and latent risks that victims of strangulation can experience. Nursing knowledge of the signs and symptoms of strangulation along with assessment tools that allow for comprehensive clinical evaluation are essential for optimizing outcomes for victims. Clinical care must be combined with support after discharge. Forensic nurses must be prepared to offer resources to victims of strangulation to decrease risks of lethal outcomes. Interdisciplinary and external partnerships with agents dedicated to the support of victims of IPV can increase the effectiveness of care for victims of strangulation.

RESOURCES

Non-Fatal Strangulation Documentation Toolkit. Retrieved from https://c.ymcdn.com/sites/iafn.siteym.com/resource/resmgr/resources/Strangulation_Documentation_.pdf

The National Domestic Violence Hotline. Retrieved from http://www.thehotline.org

Facts Victims of Strangulation (Choking) Need to Know Brochure. Retrieved from https://www.familyjusticecenter.org/resources/facts-victims-strangulation-choking-need-know-brochure

Training Institute on Strangulation Prevention: Brochures-English and Spanish. Retrieved from https://www.strangulationtraining-institute.com/resources/library/brochures-english-spanish

References

Funk, M., & Schuppel, J. (2003). Strangulation injuries. *Wisconsin Medical Journal, 102*(3), 41–45.

Glass, N., Laughon, K., Campbell, J., Wolf-Chair, A. D., Block, C. R., Hanson, G., Sharps, P. W., & Taliaferro, E. (2008). *Journal of Emergency Medicine, 35*(3), 329–335. doi:10.1018/jeremermed.2007.02.065

Pritchard, A. J., Reckdenwald, A., & Nordham, C. (2017). Non-fatal strangulation as part of domestic violence: A review of research. *Trauma, Violence & Abuse,* 18(4), 407–424. doi:10.1177/1524838015622439

Scannell, M., MacDonald, A. E., & Foster, C. (2017). Strangulation: What every nurse must recognize. *Nursing Made Incredibly Easy, 15,* 41–46. doi:10.1097/01.NME.00005255552.06539.02

Sorenson, S. B., Joshi, M., & Sivitx, E. (2014). A systematic review of the epidemiology of non-fatal strangulation: A human rights and health concern. *American Journal of Public Health, 104*(11), 54–61. doi:10.2105/AJPH.2014.302191

United States Preventative Task Force. (2013). *Screening for intimate partner violence and abuse of the elderly.* Retrieved from http://www.uspreventativeservicestaskforce.org/Home/GetFileByID/1891

15

Human Trafficking

Andrea MacDonald

Human trafficking (HT) is an insidious and traumatic crime against humanity. Healthcare providers, particularly emergency department (ED) providers, have been identified as those most likely to interact with HT victims during exploitation. Comprehensive education about the signs and symptoms of HT, including identification of high-risk populations and screening/ treatment modalities, is an important provision for healthcare providers. Nurses are often the first providers to interact with patients in healthcare settings. HT education for nurses must be prioritized to create the dynamic collaboration within the healthcare system that is necessary to eradicate HT.

This chapter provides an overview of HT by describing victimology/vulnerable populations, possible scenarios, and victim presentations. The signs and symptoms of HT are also described with a special focus on "red flag" indicators. Treatment of victims, including trauma-informed care (TIC) practices and safety planning for special circumstances, are discussed. Resources for aftercare are also described.

At the end of this chapter, the nurse will be able to:

1. Recognize populations at a high risk for HT.
2. Identify the signs and symptoms of HT.

3. Provide focused treatment to victims of HT, including safety planning.
4. Identify resources and services that victims of HT can access for support/assistance.

BACKGROUND

The U.S. Department of State (2012) defines "human trafficiking" as "the act of recruiting, harboring, transporting, providing or obtaining a person for compelled labor or commercial sex acts using fraud, force or coercion" (Byrne, Parish, & Ghilain, 2017). There has been documentation of HT in nearly all countries and all industries. Forms of HT include labor trafficking, sex trafficking, and organ/tissue trafficking, with labor trafficking being the most common form of trafficking at the global level. HT is estimated to be an industry of US\$32 billion per year (DeLay & Byrne, 2016; Trossman, 2008), though this may be a conservative figure given the covert nature of HT, as this illegal activity often remains undiscovered (Grace, Ahn, & Macias-Kontantopoulos, 2014). Individuals of all ages, genders, and races are affected by HT, meaning the scope of the problem is broad. Despite global legislation criminalizing HT, it is believed that more individuals are in forced servitude today than during the slave trade of the 19th century (Trout, 2010). In 2010, Germany was ranked first in global commerce for HT, with the United States ranking a close second (Dovydaitis, 2010). Females make up the majority of HT victims at 55% of the total victim pool. Of the 11.4 million females who are victimized, they represent nearly all of the 22% of victims who are sexually exploited and also represent approximately 40% of forced labor exploitation victims. Children are thought to represent 26% of all HT victims (CdeBaca & Sigmon, 2014; Dovydaitis, 2010).

The average time of exploitation for labor-trafficked victims is 18 months (CdeBaca & Sigmon, 2014). There are no reliable statistics on the time of incarceration for sex-trafficked victims (Alvarez, 2016). Clearly, the conditions of HT contribute to negative health consequences, which typically result in victims accessing the healthcare system, though access is often limited and sporadic. A skilled assessment and the care of HT victims is critical for nurses due to the limited opportunities to assist victims with freedom, recovery, and restoration of wellness.

AT-RISK POPULATIONS

Although HT is seen in all demographics, certain populations are particularly vulnerable to victimization. Lack of resources has been directly linked to HT as individuals who cannot provide for themselves and who perceive themselves to lack support systems are at higher risk for HT (Jani & Anstadt, 2013; Kiss, Yun, Pocock, & Zimmerman, 2015; Konstantopoulos et al., 2015). These individuals include (but are not limited to):

- Homeless individuals
- Runaways
- Those growing up in families or environments with violence: abuse, neglect, domestic violence
- Undocumented individuals
- Minors under the age of 18
- Limited education
- Members of the lesbian, gay, bisexual, transgender, queer/questioning, and intersex (LGBTQI)
- Individuals with substance addiction/abuse issues
- Financially unstable individuals
- Individuals with mental illness
- Intellectually challenged individuals
- Immigrants from developed countries (Panagabutra-Roberts, 2012)

ROLE OF THE FORENSIC NURSE AND "RED FLAGS" FOR HT

Nurses are in a prime position to screen, identify, treat, and refer victims of HT (Association of Women's Health, Obstetrics and Neonatal Nurses, 2016). There is a multitude of barriers to detection of HT, even to expert providers. There is not a single element or combination thereof that can determine HT with full certainty (Schwartz et al., 2016). The signs listed have been determined to be red flags that should prompt more intense assessment. The final sign is "branding," the act of permanently marking a victim. Traffickers often use permanent or temporary tattoos (some conventional ink and others less conventional such as cutting or scarring) to designate "ownership" of the victim. A crown, name, or initials placed in a prominent place (face, chest, neck) of the victim should warrant concern for HT (Peters, 2013; Sabella, 2011).

Fast Facts

Signs and symptoms of human trafficking can be difficult to detect by healthcare providers during a typically brief-interaction visit. Victims seldom self-identify and often present with a medical condition that might not seem to be directly related to imprisonment or coercion.

Some of the key signs and symptoms of HT are listed below (Polaris Project, n.d.; Sabella, 2011):

- Victim is not allowed to speak to healthcare provider alone or someone else is answering for them.
- Victim does not have access to important personal documents (license/passport/bank account).
- Victim is hesitant or unable to answer questions about his or her health condition or living situation/employment.
- Victim seems unusually fearful/paranoid regarding healthcare providers and/or law enforcement.
- Victim's healthcare concern is not consistent with presentation for care.
- Victim's age is not consistent with appearance.
- Victim has a tattoo/marking that he or she cannot/will not explain (branding ; Peters, 2013).
- Victim has a disheveled appearance, poor hygiene, or clothes not appropriate for the weather.

POSSIBLE CLINICAL PRESENTATIONS FOR HT VICTIMS

HT victims can present with any complaint. Many victims have chronic medical conditions such as diabetes or hypertension that may go untreated while being exploited. These victims may present with commonly seen conditions such as elevated blood sugar or chest pain. Detection of HT in this type of presentation requires expert knowledge of the more subtle signs and symptoms of HT that may be elicited during the full nursing assessment. HT victims may present with trauma or strain injuries related to labor trafficking or head/neck/oral trauma related to sex trafficking. Organ trafficking victims may have very obvious traumatic/emergency injuries such as blood loss, infection, or evisceration. Some more common clinical presentations for HT victims are:

- Untreated or poorly controlled medical conditions: diabetes, hypertension, HIV
- Sexually transmitted infections
- Reproductive problems: miscarriage, preterm labor, septic abortions, pregnancy testing
- Genitourinary and rectal problems: incontinence and infections
- Injuries related to strangulation: head/neck/oral/auricular problems
- Lacerations, burns, or fractures that are acute or in different stages of healing
- Head injuries from trauma

- Defensive wounds, located on back of arms
- Respiratory conditions related to suboptimal environmental conditions
- Malnutrition, dehydration, and dental problems related to a lack of nutrition
- Presence of infectious diseases (e.g., tuberculosis [TB]) that have been eradicated
- Complications of substance use, overdose, drug addiction, or drug-seeking behaviors
- Acute mental health crisis, posttraumatic stress disorder, or suicidality

CASE STUDIES

Case 1: Vicky

Vicky is a 24-year-old female who was brought to the ED by the emergency medical services (EMS) after she was found unresponsive next to a radiator at a drug detox facility. On EMS arrival, she received 4 mg of nasal Narcan, became conscious, and was taken to the ED. Past medical history includes hepatitis C, pancreatitis, asthma, gastritis, and pelvic inflammatory disease. Past mental health history includes anxiety, depression, posttraumatic stress disorder, bipolar affective disorder, and a suicide attempt. When she was responsive, she reported her boyfriend followed her to the drug detox facility and dragged her into the bathroom where he injected her with heroin. He then tried to carry her out of the facility but was unable to lift her. She was left lying unconscious next to the radiator.

The ED visit consisted of a comprehensive assessment with cardiac monitoring and an extended stay in the ED observation unit for ongoing assessment. She had sustained a second-degree burn to her shoulder and a sterile dressing was applied. She was started on antibiotics for pneumonia and potential sexually transmitted infections. Upon stabilization, Vicky reported that her boyfriend forced her to have sex with strangers for money that was then used to pay for drugs. A sexual assault nurse examiner (SANE) evaluation was offered but Vicky declined. Vicky was living with her boyfriend and requested assistance with placement in safe housing. She remained in the observation unit for several hours and was discharged to a rehabilitation facility. Follow-up care was scheduled for HT-related concerns.

Case 2: Kim

Kim is a 35-year-old female who presented to the ED with a chief complaint of diabetic ketoacidosis (DKA). More than 20 hours into her visit, Kim disclosed sexual assault and HT. Kim's trafficker was her boss with whom she originally had a consensual romantic relationship and shared a home. When Kim tried to end the relationship, her trafficker threatened to ruin her reputation and earning capability in her profession (Kim worked as a plumber). Kim endured ongoing domestic violence, sexual assault by the trafficker, and threats to her life. Her past medical history included type I diabetes mellitus, DKA, asthma, migraines, childhood sexual abuse, and sexual assault. Past mental health history included anxiety, depression, and posttraumatic stress disorder. Kim had a history of homelessness in the past and had lived with three children and an elderly relative affected by dementia prior to moving in with her trafficker. She had a history of involvement with the Department of Children and Family Services (DCFS) due to a history of domestic violence. She also reported daily marijuana use.

Kim's ED course consisted of treatment of her DKA, which required admission to the medical intensive care unit (MICU). Kim was stabilized and transferred to the medical floor prior to discharge to home. During her admission, Kim was referred to a specialized aftercare clinic for survivors of sexual assault and HT. Kim was provided with resources and was able to move forward and escape her trafficker. She remains employed in her trade and is living independently at present (Scannell, MacDonald, Berger, & Boyer, 2018).

FORENSIC NURSING IMPLICATIONS

Implications for forensic nursing include creating and disseminating evidence-based and research-informed practice and knowledge related to HT across disciplines in order to improve recognition and enhance treatment. Forensic nursing is grounded in biology, psychology, social ethics, and spirituality. Forensic nurses must educate all nurses in how to diagnose and treat individuals and groups who have been affected by violence and trauma. An integrative approach that utilizes forensic and nursing processes is essential to creating successful treatment plans that support the restoration of optimal wellness for victims.

A unique aspect of forensic nursing is its foundation in both social and legal processes. Forensic nurses not only provide expert care but also collect evidence for forensic analysis. The highest level of awareness of the health and legal consequences is paramount to forensic nursing practice. Evidence can be used to influence and create social policy as well as to support legal processes, such as the incarceration of traffickers. The American Nurses Association and the International Association of Forensic Nurses both endorse the view that forensic nursing is the intersection between health and legal systems given that forensic nurses must be attentive to the medical, psychosocial, spiritual, and legal needs of their patients. Advocacy must extend to guidance of other members of the multidisciplinary care team who may not have a background in forensic practice. The forensic nurse must lead the team to ensure that maximum standards of health assessment, expert specimen collection for forensic analysis, proper legal standards of reporting, and optimal posthospital support services are in place for all victims of HT.

Forensic nursing is distinctive in many ways, particularly as it is focused on populations affected by violence and trauma. Practice is not limited to episodic treatment but extends globally in the form of impacts on local, regional, and global health practices and policy. Forensic nursing requires an integrative approach that includes a science/evidence-based nursing practice along with collaboration across multiple practice environments including medicine, law, politics, psychology, and spiritual agencies. The success of forensic nursing efforts toward victim wellness and recovery is contingent upon a continuous collaborative practice that must have a wide global reach.

TREATMENT AND RESOURCES

Treatment of HT requires a multifaceted approach that is guided by the principles of TIC. All life-threatening conditions, such as physical trauma or sepsis, must be addressed as a priority. When physical safety has been established, healthcare providers must proceed on the care continuum toward establishing a trusting relationship, which is critical to creating a therapeutic relationship between patient and providers.

Fast Facts

TIC is a sensitive approach to address the unique psychological circumstances of trauma that may impact the ability of a victim to engage productively in effective self-care.

A standardized trauma assessment process should be used to guide medical care and should be followed by screening for HT. Several standardized screening tools can be used to assess for HT risk/involvement. When HT is detected, care must be problem-focused. Victims should be treated for safety, as well as medical, social, financial, and spiritual concerns. Treatment of HT victims must be interdisciplinary and extend beyond the initial healthcare visit.

Collaboration between healthcare disciplines such as social work, nursing, and medicine must occur to create effective discharge plans. Coordination of services with external agencies is a benchmark that healthcare agencies must achieve in order to provide comprehensive care for HT victims. HT victims are at the highest risk of harm, including death, during the process of escaping a trafficking situation, so treatment plans must include safety planning. This requires resources that can be accessed by the victim upon discharge from the healthcare setting. The following list offers links to HT screening tools and resources that can be accessed by healthcare providers to assist victims of HT in moving toward recovery.

Fast Facts

Victim identification is the first step toward victim recovery and eradication of human trafficking as a crime against humanity.

CONCLUSION

HT remains an underidentified and underreported healthcare and social crisis. Barriers to recognition include a lack of research, a lack of provider education, the inability of victims to self-identify, and a lack of resources (Chisolm-Straker, Richardson, & Cossio, 2012). An accurate understanding of the signs and symptoms of HT along with an awareness of at-risk populations will enable healthcare providers to assess and treat victims properly so they can move toward recovery. Provider access to screening tools and hospital- and community-based resources for victims promotes the ability to deliver highly effective patient-centered care. Healthcare providers can lead the movement to eradicate HT so that social health and wellness are promoted. Commitment to "looking below the surface" is the key to increasing the detection of HT (U.S. Department of State, 2013). The eradication of HT is an ethical mandate that all healthcare providers must champion.

RESOURCES

HT Screening Tool Links

Comprehensive Human Trafficking Assessment Tool. Retrieved from https://humantraffickinghotline.org/resources/comprehensive-human-trafficking-assessment-tool

U.S. Department of Health and Human Services Screening Tool for Victims of Human Trafficking. Retrieved from https://www.acf.

hhs.gov/sites/default/files/orr/screening_questions_to_assess_
whether_a_person_is_a_trafficking_victim_0.pdf

Vera Institute of Justice—A Tool for the Identification of Human Trafficking. Retrieved from https://www.vera.org/publications/out-of-
the-shadows-identification-of-victims-of-human-trafficking

HT Victim Agency Resources

U.S. Department of Health and Human Services
Administration for Children and Families
Campaign to Rescue and Restore Victims of Human Trafficking
1-888-373-7888
www.acf.hhs.gov/trafficking

Catholic Charities Community Services
Developing Individual Growth and New Independence Through
    Yourself (DIGNITY)
www.catholiccharitiesaz.org/catholiccharities/dignity.aspx

Coalition Against Trafficking in Women
www.catwinternational.org

Free the Slaves
www.freetheslaves.net

Humantrafficking.org
www.humantrafficking.org

Local Law Enforcement
911 or local contact number

Polaris Project
www.polarisproject.org

Stop the Traffik
www.stopthetraffik.org

The Office for Victims of Crime
1-800-672-6872

References

Alvarez, P. (2016). When sex trafficking goes unnoticed in America.
    Retrieved from http://www.theatlantic.com/politics/archive/2016/02/
    when-sex-trafficking-goes-unnoticed-in-America/470166

Association of Women's Health, Obstetrics and Neonatal Nurses. (2016). Human trafficking: AWHOON position statement. *Journal of Obstetric, Gynecological & Neonatal Nursing, 45*(3), 458–460. doi:10.1016/j. ogn.2016.04.001

Byrne, M., Parish, B., & Ghilain, C. (2017). Victims of human trafficking: Hiding in plain sight. *Nursing, 47*(3), 48–52. doi:10.1097/01. NURSE.0000512876.06634.c4

CdeBaca, L., & Sigmon, J. N. (2014). Combating trafficking in persons: A call to action for global health professionals. *Global Health: Science & Practice, 2*(3), 261–267. doi:10.9745/GHSP-D-13-00142

Chisolm-Straker, M., Richardson, L. D., & Cossio, T. (2012). Combating slavery in the 21st Century: The role of emergency medicine. *Journal of Healthcare for the Poor and Under-served, 23*, 980–987. doi:10.1353/ hpu.2012.0091

DeLay, J., & Byrne, M. (2016). How nurses can make a difference: Recognizing victims of human trafficking. *Imprint, 63*, 43–45.

Dovydaitis, T. (2010). Human trafficking: The role of the health care provider. *Journal of Midwifery & Women's Health, 55*(5), 462–467. doi:10.1016/j. jmwh.2009.12.017

Grace, A. M., Ahn, R., & Macias-Kontantopoulos, W. (2014). Integrating curricula on human trafficking into medical education and residency training. *Journal of American Medical Association in Pediatrics, 168*(9), 793–794. doi:10.1001/jamapediatrics.2014.999

Jani, N., & Anstadt, S. P. (2013). Contributing factors in trafficking from south Asia. *Journal of Human Behavior in the Social Environment, 23*(3), 298–311. doi:10.1097/TME0000000000000138

Kiss, L., Yun, K., Pocock, N., & Zimmerman, C. (2015). Exploitation, violence, and suicide risk among child and adolescent survivors of human trafficking in the greater Mekong subregion. *Journal of the American Medical Association in Pediatrics, 169*(9), e152278. doi:10.1001/ jamapediatrics.2015.2278

Konstantopoulos, W. M., Munroe, D., Purcell, G., Tester, K., Burke, T. F., & Ahn, R. (2015). The commercial sexual exploitation and sex trafficking of minors in the Boston metropolitan area: Experiences and challenges faced by front-line providers and other stakeholders. *Journal of Applied Research on Children: Informing Policy for Children at Risk, 6*(1), 1–26.

Panagabutra-Roberts, A. (2012). Human trafficking in the United States: Part 1: State of the knowledge. *Behavioral & Social Sciences Librarian, 31*(3), 138–151. doi:10.1080/01639269.2012.736330

Peters, K. (2013). The growing business of human trafficking and the power of emergency nurses to stop it. *Journal of Emergency Nursing, 39*(3), 280–288. doi:10.1016/j.jen.201203.017

Polaris Project. (n.d.). Recognize the signs. Retrieved from https://polaris-project.org/human-trafficking/recognize-signs

Sabella, D. (2011). The role of the nurse in combating human trafficking. *American Journal of Nursing, 111*(2), 28–37. doi:10.1097/01. NAJ.0000394289.555.b6

Scannell, M., MacDonald, A. E., Berger, A., & Boyer, N. (2018). Human trafficking: How nurses can make a difference. *Journal of Forensic Nursing, 14*(2), 117–121. doi:10.1097/JFN.0000000000000203

Schwartz, C., Unruh, E., Cronin, K., Evans-Simpson, S., Britton, H., & Ramaswamy, M. (2016). Human trafficking identification and service provision in the medical and social services sectors. *Health & Human Rights Journal, 18*(1), 181–192.

Trossman, S. (2008). The costly business of human trafficking. *American Nurse Today, 3*(12). Retrieved from http://www.americannursetoday.com/the-costly-business-of-human-trafficking

Trout, K. K. (2010). The role of nurses in identifying and helping victims of human trafficking. *Pennsylvania Nurse, 5*(4), 18–20.

U.S. Department of State. (2012). *Trafficking in persons report 2012.* Retrieved from https://www.state.gov/j/tip/rls/tiprpt/2012/192352.htm

U.S. Department of State. (2013). Victim identification: The first step in stopping modern slavery. *Trafficking in persons report 2013.* Retrieved from https://www.state.gov/j/tip/rls/tiprpt/2013/210542.htm

16

Gunshot Wounds

Meredith J. Scannell

Gunshot wounds (GSWs), intentional and nonintentional, have a significant impact on the health of individuals and greatly impact society at large and healthcare costs in the United States. Victims of GSWs can be found in various settings, and forensic nurses and others may be caring for victims in a variety of settings, including wound assessments, evidence collection, or even death investigation. Having an understanding of the impact GSWs have can help address this serious public health problem.

At the end of the chapter, the nurse will be able to:

1. Identify the different types of firearms and types of injuries they can inflict.
2. List the process of evidence collation in regards to GSWs.
3. Understand the necessary aspects of mandatory reporting.

BACKGROUND

GSWs are an epidemic problem in the Unites states and globally, impacting the health and lives of individuals. GSWs are one of the leading causes of deaths in the United States. The rates of death from GSWs vary from state to state. In 2016, Massachusetts was the lowest at 3.4 per 100,000 population and Alaska the highest at 23.3 per

100,000 population (National Center for Health Statistics, 2018). The leading causes of GSW death are suicide, homicide, unintentional, and legal intervention such as law enforcement and military and last nondeterminate (Murphy et al., 2017).

TYPES OF FIREARMS

There are numerous types of firearms, ranging from low to high velocity. Handguns are considered low velocity, and the projectile can be a single bullet from a handheld pistol or multiple bullets from a semiautomatic pistol. Shotguns are considered high velocity and fire a mass of pellets and are very destructive at close range. There are also many types of bullets with different tips and markings. The caliber refers to the diameter of the bullet.

TISSUE DAMAGE

Damage to tissue from a gunshot depends on the type of firearm, bullet, distance range, and kinetic energy that is deposited into the tissue. The types of tissue injuries from bullets include laceration, crushing injuries, cavitation, and shock waves. Some bullets leave entrance and exit wounds, while others leave an entrance wound and no exit wound. Tissue and bones that are in the path of the bullet are injured. A GSW leaves a permanent cavity and entrance wound, which is the size of the bullet, and often appears as a circular mark with blackened edges that have seared. Some bullets enter the body with such force and velocity that they stretch and tear surrounding tissue. A stellate shape can occur when gas enters the point of entry and stretches out over the skin. Different tissues and organs within the body have different levels of susceptibility to energy, causing greater harm and injury from the bullet. Wounds from a gunshot can have various other markings on the skin. Gunshot residue is burnt gunpowder that can give a soot appearance on the skin surrounding the entrance wound. Tattooing occurs when the gunpowder embeds into the skin surrounding the entrance wound. Entrance wounds are often smaller and more irregular in appearance than exit wounds and can have a slit-like or stellate appearance. Exit wounds are often irregular and larger than entrance wounds and may or may not have a straight path from the entrance wound, as some bullets may tumble and veer off the straight path as they make contact with the body and lose energy (Rhee et al., 2016).

Fast Facts

It is important not to assume or document entrance and exit wounds, as the assumption can be wrong and this can have legal implications.

Thing to consider when examining someone with a GSW:

- Was the gunshot due to an accident, suicide attempt, or intentional violence?
- What type of weapon was used?
- What was the range of distance?

First always treat any life-threatening wound and stabilize the patient prior to completing a wound assessment. If the patient is stable, you can evaluate, document, and collect forensic evidence prior to treating the wound. All wounds should be evaluated and documented separately, including their physical features (size, shape) and surrounding markings. A body traumagram should be used to indicate where on the body the wounds were found. The wounds from a gunshot vary depending on the range of contact, such as close, medium, or long range. Photographs should be taken according to hospital policy and according to Health Insurance Portability and Accountability Act of 1996 (HIPAA) policy using standard forensic techniques of photographing close- and long-range picture and using a standard object or a measuring device, such as a ruler, in the photographs. Photographs should first be taken as the patient presents to the hospital and then again after cleaning any debris, soot, or blood from the skin. The local police department can take the photographs as evidence with consent from the patient.

EVIDENCE COLLECTION

In cases of GSWs there may be a need to identify, collect, and preserve forensic evidence. It is important to follow the hospital policy and local law regarding samples required by law enforcement. A chain of custody must be maintained and documented to preserve the integrity of the evidence.

Bullets

If bullets are retrieved out of the patient, they should be collected for evidence. Bullets have unique characteristics and markings that can identify the weapon used in the shooting and eliminate suspects. Bullets should not be handled with metal instruments such as metal forceps, as this risks the potential of making marks or scrapes on the bullet, which can have legal implications. The bullet should be placed on a sterile 4 × 4 gauze without removing any debris and placed into a sterile container with holes on the top of the container to allow for ventilation and to prevent the bullet from rusting. All bullets must be placed in their own individual containers with the patient's name on each container, along with medical record number, location of where the bullet was found, and the name of the person who removed it (Masteller et al., 2014).

Clothing

All clothing should be preserved for forensic evidence, as there can be gun residue that can help determine the range of the shot and the entrance/exit wounds (Snow & Bozeman, 2010). In cases where clothing needs to be cut off the patient, it is essential to cut around the bullet holes to preserve evidence. If it is unavoidable to cut around the bullet hole, then documentations should indicate that a cut was made. All clothing should be placed in an individual paper bag with the patient's name, medical record number, and item of clothing. Plastic bags should be avoided at all cost, as environmental factors can degrade the evidence.

Fingertips

There may be a need to gather evidence from the patient's fingertips. Gunpowder and primer residue may be on the fingers of the patient especially if he or she was the one who pulled the trigger of the gun. The presence or absence of gunpowder on the individual's hand can indicate the intent of the gunshot: suicide versus homicide (Snow & Bozeman, 2010).

OTHER TREATMENTS TO CONSIDER

If a patient does present for care after a GSW, he or she should have a thorough examination with clothing removed to assess for any other injuries or GSWs. X-rays can be helpful to identify the location of the bullets and to determine if more bullets are present. All patients with GSWs should have prophylactic antibiotics to prevent infection. GSWs are considered contaminated as the bullet can introduce external material such as clothing, skin, and hair into the body upon entrance. The tetanus status of the patient should be determined, and the patient should be given vaccination if it is not up to date.

Prevention

Nurses in all healthcare settings can be instrumental in addressing prevention efforts related to gun control. At all healthcare visits, asking about gun safety and access to guns should be part of universal screening. This will help identify those at higher risk for gun injuries and how safety measures can be implemented to help reduce accidental and intentional GSWs.

Mandatory Reporting

Most states have mandatory reporting laws about how GSWs must be reported to the jurisdictional law enforcement when the injury occurred. This includes cases of self-harm and accidental injuries.

CONCLUSION

Gun injuries have a devastating effect on the lives of individuals and communities at large. Knowing the evidence-based practice in evidence collection and wound identification can help determine the cause of the GSW and help to provide linkage to appropriate resources and services. Nurses can be instrumental in addressing gun safety by screening for unsafe gun practices or access and can help mitigate gun injuries, both intentional and unintentional. Having an understanding of who is at risk can help focus efforts in prevention and safety.

References

Masteller, M. A., Prahlow, A., Walsh, M. M., Thomas, S. G., Wolfenbarger, R., & Prahlow, J. A. (2014). Proper handling of bullet evidence in trauma patients. *Trauma, 16*(3), 189–194. doi:10.1177/1460408614532047

Murphy, S. L., Xu, J. Q., Kochanek, K. D., Curtin, S. C., & Arias, E. (2017). Deaths: Final data for 2015. *National Vital Statistics Reports, 66*(6). Hyattsville, MD: National Center for Health Statistics.

National Center for Health Statistics. (2018). Firearm mortality by state. Retrieved from https://www.cdc.gov/nchs/pressroom/sosmap/firearm_mortality/firearm.htm

Rhee, P. M., Moore, E. E., Joseph, B., Tang, A., Pandit, V., & Vercruysse, G. (2016). Gunshot wounds: A review of ballistics, bullets, weapons, and myths. *Journal of Trauma and Acute Care Surgery, 80*(6), 853–867. doi:10.1097/TA.0000000000001037

Snow, A., & Bozeman, J. (2010). Role implications for nurses caring for gunshot wound victims. *Critical Care Nursing Quarterly, 33*(3), 259–264. doi:10.1097/CNQ.0b013e3181e65fec

17

Acts of Terrorism: Healthcare in the Age of Modern Terrorism

Yaeko Marie Karantonis

Acts of terrorism are not a new occurrence in the world or even in the United States. Healthcare providers have always provided treatment to victims of violence; the act of caring for victims of terrorism carries an extended burden. The likelihood of caring for a victim of a terrorist event has increased over recent years, which has resulted in the necessity to employ additional information and training into practice. Forensic nursing has an important role in the care of this population. The forensic nurse must use his or her training to aid in the identification of a terror event, provide care safely to the injured, and assist with the social and legal ramifications of a terrorist incident. Presented in this chapter are personal experiences of healthcare professionals responding to the victims of the 2013 Boston Marathon bombing.

Upon completion of this chapter, the nurse will be able to:

1. Identify an act of terrorism.
2. Implement an awareness of potential personal safety and security considerations.
3. Recognize the role of responders in aiding the legal system.

BACKGROUND

In 1794, during the French Revolution, the term *terrorisme* was used in regard to the rule of the Jacobin faction troops as a pejorative label. The idea of terrorism originates in 1869 from Sergey Nechayev, a Russian revolutionary, who used the term to describe himself. Nechayev believed the pursuit of his beliefs was necessary by any means. At this time in history, there is no globally agreed upon singular definition of "terrorism" due to the political and emotional implications injected into the term. Even within a single government, there can be multiple definitions of terrorism. The North Atlantic Treaty Organization (NATO) defines "terrorism" as "[t]he unlawful use or threatened use of force or violence, instilling fear and terror, against individuals or property in an attempt to coerce or intimidate governments or societies, or to gain control over a population, to achieve political, religious or ideological objectives" (International Military Staff, 2016, Terrorism).

In recent history, there have been multiple terrorist events. In 2017 alone, there were over 100 incidents of terrorism reported monthly throughout the world (National Consortium for the Study of Terrorism and Responses to Terrorism (START), 2018).

Listed are a few events that have occurred in the past 30 years:

- Ted Kaczynski/Unabomber 1978–1995 (multiple locations)
- Rajneeshee bioterror attack in Dalles, Oregon, 1984
- Alfred P. Murrah Federal Building bombing, Oklahoma City, Oklahoma, 1995
- Tokyo subway sarin attack, Tokyo, Japan, 1995
- Centennial Olympic Park bombing, Atlanta, Georgia, 1996
- World Trade Center, New York City, New York, 2001
- Anthrax mailing, Washington, DC, 2001
- Beltway Sniper shootings, 2002
- Boston Marathon bombing, Boston, Massachusetts, 2013
- Charleston Church shooting, Charleston, South Carolina, 2015

Historically, terrorism has been perpetrated with chemical, biological, radiological, nuclear, and explosive/munitions (CBRNE) weapons. Now, there is a growing use of cyber technologies as a means of terrorism. Cyberterrorism has been reported or suspected in recent attacks on Estonia in 2007 and an attack during the U.S. presidential elections of 2016. Due to this, there is increased attention to the role of cyberterrorism, which can impact infrastructure and industry.

Due to the advent of the Internet and social media, the proliferation of ideas and causes are not as isolated as they once were. Terror groups have become adept at identifying and recruiting new members by using social media marketing. Worldwide recruiting can now be done from one's living room. Propaganda videos attempt to appeal to young people through methods such as promoting a "jihad cool" sentiment to influence and indoctrinate them. Terrorist groups are no longer restricted by a physical location; membership can now be expansive throughout the world (Huey, 2015).

Fast Facts

Despite having over 100 different interpretations of terrorism, the definitive sentiment remains the same throughout all definitions. It is the purpose of an act that is perpetrated on a population or property with the intent to evoke harm, fear, chaos, and/or disruption in an attempt to influence or support politics, religions, or ideologies. Terrorism can be executed by many means, including the use of CBRNE and cyberattacks.

SAFETY AND SECURITY

The goal of terrorist attacks is to interrupt the normal activities of a society and bring about as much panic and alarm as possible. The concern for secondary attacks or devices is always a worry. Reported attacks constructed to disable investigators, first responders, and healthcare responders have been suspected in attacks such as the 2002 Bali bombings and the 1997 Atlanta Olympic Park bombings. Personal safety must always be a consideration during a terror attack. The lack of knowledge of the weapon, the number of weapons, and intention of the terrorist often can make normal behaviors risky (Thompson, Rehn, Lossius, & Lockey, 2014).

During the Boston Marathon in 2013, two explosions occurred. The eruptions occurred approximately 13 seconds and 180 feet apart. The type and construct of the device were not known when the incident occurred (Project Management Team, 2014). As the first explosion occurred, many unknowingly ran toward the area where the second explosion occurred. Hundreds were injured, many losing their limbs, and three were killed (Gates et al., 2014). A mass casualty response ensued with transport of the critically injured to local hospitals. A false account of another device was reported near the location of ambulance staging (Jill Brown, personal communication, November 15, 2017).

Personal protection equipment (PPE) is a concept with which those who work in the healthcare industry are acquainted; staff routinely dons gloves, gowns, masks, and eye shields when caring for patients. Precaution is taken with bodily fluids, sharp items, and potential communicable diseases. In dealing with a victim of violence, there is awareness of a potential ongoing threat to the victim and a potential weapon risk (Blank-Reid & Bokholdt, 2014). All of these practices must be employed in dealing with victims of terror-ism. Many victims of violence are targeted and carry some level of prediction or cause. Victims of terrorism differ in this respect. It is not the individual who is the focus but rather what the person(s) rep-resents to the attacker. In addition, the act of terrorism is to inflict harm or distress on as many people as possible.

Weapons of terrorism are varied and can be expansive. More than one weapon can be used in an attack and there can be more than one target. This must always be considered when involved in a response to a terrorist attack. Scene training focuses on personal safety over victim care. This focus on personal safety must extend to secondary care sites such as morgues, hospitals, and clinics that provide care to the victims. This concept goes against many healthcare providers' instincts to provide quick care to victims.

The Boston Marathon's first bomb exploded at 2:49 p.m. The sources of the explosions were initially unknown. Hospitals were notified 4 minutes after the first bomb exploded and were informed that two explosions had occurred near the densely crowded mara-thon finish line. The on-site ambulances started to transport patients to local hospitals prior to any assessment reports of contamination at the scene. Some facilities did not receive any other information prior to the arrival of patients. The average time from explosion to initial arrival at hospitals was 11 minutes. At 3:00 p.m. (11 minutes after the first explosion), no detection of chemical or radiological substances related to the bombs was found at the scene, but this information was not communicated to receiving hospitals. Hospitals were receiving unknown numbers of critically ill patients with an unknown con-tamination status (Project Management Team, 2014).

In a short time, multiple patients and employees began arriving at the hospitals with no effective effort to control entry points to the hospital or emergency room. The arrivals were not searched for weapons. In at least one instance, a hospital received a potential per-petrator of the attack, but the person was not searched prior to entry into the hospital.

In response to this incident, many healthcare workers did not employ the added requirement for personal safety. The focus was delivering care for those who were severely injured and had lost their limbs. Upon the victims entering the hospital, without knowledge of any contamination assessments, staff members became poten-tial victims of an exposure (Centers for Diseases Control and Pre-vention, 2018). Lack of effective security measures allowed the flow of unknown persons into the facility and also lacked proper con-sideration for additional weapons on persons entering. There was no contamination exposure to staff due to the attack, and there were no reported incidents of additional terrorist activity at the hospital (Jodi Swenson, personal communication, October 6, 2017). The Boston healthcare workers are not alone in this focus of providing care over personal safety.

The sarin attack by the Aum Shinrikyo cult in the Tokyo subway system in 1995 also presented challenges for the staff in Tokyo. On the first day of the incident, St. Luke's Hospital received 640 patients and a total of 1,410 patients over the next 7 days. Similar to what occurred in Boston, the hospital quickly became overwhelmed with patients and persons entering the hospital. A gas explosion was initially reported as the cause of the mass casualty incident. The staff was unaware that the substance affecting the arriving patients was actually the chemical nerve agent sarin, and they were wearing PPE that was inadequate against such a chemical. As a result, it was reported that 245 healthcare workers associated with the Tokyo incident developed symptoms that can be attributed to sarin exposure (Okumura et al., 1998).

Both the Boston and Tokyo incidents demonstrate a need for integrating a stronger practice of personal protection and safety during a terrorist attack. The first step to improve the protection of persons is to recognize the potential of the event as a terror attack. Many of us in school were taught the five Ws: What, Who, Why, When, Where.

FIVE Ws

1. **WHAT** happened? Is this a natural/normal event? Could it be sinister?
2. **WHO** are these people? Could they represent anything? Who is the instigator?
3. **WHY** did this occur? Could it be ideologically/politically motivated?
4. **WHEN** did this occur? Is this date or time significant?
5. **WHERE**? Is the location significant? Is there anything happening in this community?

An analysis should be done when faced with acts of violence or cases of increased numbers of persons affected. Applying these simple investigative questions can help identify an event as concerning and therefore invoke a consideration for augmenting the necessary high level of protection and security practices (American Nurses Association & International Association of Forensic Nurses, 2009).

Despite a great deal of focus on the threats of CBRNE at a terror attack scene, it is not the greatest threat to responders. The greatest secondary threat to all workers who respond to a terror attack is the scene itself. The environment may be damaged due to impact. Infrastructure may be weakened and vulnerable. The more traditional scene hazards of unstable buildings, live electrical wires, fire, building debris, and airborne particulate pose a larger danger to workers. Evidence of such secondary injury has been evidenced by the response at the World Trade Center attack. Thousands of workers sustained injuries during and after the event. Many of the workers have extended health sequelae due to the poor use of protective equipment. In addition to the physical ailments, mental health injuries have been profound in the aftermath of such events (Thompson et al., 2014).

Fast Facts

Asking the basic five Ws questions in relation to an event can trigger an attentive response. Environmental awareness and early recognition of a potential terror attack are the best defenses against secondary injury. Consciousness of potential additional assaults and incorporating alertness to security threats aid in the safer response and care of terrorism victims.

LEGAL IMPLICATIONS

Upon notification that a patient who is a victim of violence presents for treatment, the staff prepares to care for the victim(s). The immediate life-saving interventions always take precedence over the legal needs. The staff has an obligation to not only treat the patient medically but also must attend to the forensic demands. Forensic nurses have been trained in the collection and the preservation of evidence (American Nurses Association & International Association of Forensic Nursing, 2015). The importance of evidence collection is essential in a terrorist event. As discussed earlier, the nature of the event may not be clear, so the evidence collected by forensic nurses can aid investigators in determining the details of the attack. One example is the evaluation of residue from an explosive on clothing or people. This residue can help investigators identify the explosive employed. The importance of evidence collection and documentation at a terrorist event cannot be understated. The amount of evidence collected during a terror attack can be staggering (National Institute of Justice, 2000).

Response to a terrorist assault can be chaotic and fast paced. In rendering care to victims, practice should include documentation and integrate evidence protective measures. Preserving the integrity of clothing can be done by attempting to not cut through tears or bullet holes in the clothing if possible. Documentation of the location and a description of injuries can assist in recreating the event.

One of the greatest complications with evidence collection from violence is transfer or cross-contamination (Grubbs, 2014). Often during emergent trauma incidents, clothing is quickly removed and thrown aside. When removing clothing, an attempt to prevent cross-contamination by placing it on a clean sheet out of the way or in a paper bag should be attempted.

During the Boston Marathon, the hospitals quickly received numerous patients into their emergency rooms. Staff had little to no time for preparations prior to this. Nurses who were not caring for patients in trauma rooms quickly realized the lack of supplies needed to preserve evidence. In one instance, a nurse realizing the need for collection of evidence retrieved paper bags from the stock room and delivered the bags to her colleagues (Tama Baker, personal communication, January 6, 2018). This action allowed the staff to keep the contamination of valuable evidence to a minimum.

Upon placing the items of evidence in bags, an inventory list and chain of custody form is created for each bag of evidence. The documentation should include the items collected, the person identifier from whom the item was removed, date and time of collection, and the collector's name and signature. For each instance when the evidence is handed over to another person, it should be reflected on the chain of custody form with date, time, and the receiver's name and signature (Eisert et al., 2010).

Fast Facts

Documentation, preservation, and collection of evidence in an event of a terror attack are an important practice. As with all evidence, attention must be paid to the integrity of the evidence, prevention of cross-contamination, and accidental transfer. An inventory and chain of custody should be maintained throughout the transfer process. The forensic nurse practice will aid the legal process and possibly prevent future attacks by doing so.

SOCIAL AND PSYCHOLOGICAL IMPACTS

The impact of terrorism on the immediate area of injury is evident in the physical and mental state of the victims. Those involved often suffer anxiety, posttraumatic stress disorder (PTSD), and depression. There is also an additional influence on the overall society in which the terror attack occurred. Not only are the victims affected, but this impact can spread beyond the scene to others in society through the media. The use of technology such as television, the Internet, and radio can expand the psychological influence to others in remote areas. Society can feel the impact of transient stressors that can extend beyond the original scene. Those not involved in the actual event can still suffer from depression, anxiety, and stress (Holman, Garfin, & Silver, 2014). Such symptoms can affect society as a whole. The impact on an industry by an increase in missed workdays and poor work performance has been demonstrated after events of terrorism. For example, in the aftermath of 9/11, people's anxiety increased regarding flying and future attacks. This increase led to less flights being purchased, and the airline industry was impacted financially, leading to layoffs. This in turn added to the emotional and psychological toll from the terrorist attack itself.

An increase in symbolic racism has been seen after a terror attack. Fear and hatred toward the perpetrators of the assault can be displaced on those who project similarities (Goodwin, Kaniasty, Sun, & Ben-Ezra, 2017). Communities can turn against their own innocent members. This distrust and paranoia can degrade communication among the population. The fissure that is created can fracture a community and, at times, a country. Although this is not as visually apparent as many types of terrorist attacks, this influence that weakens a society is nonetheless a result of terrorism. The effect on the population is the target. Terrorism is not just the "event" but also the aftermath and the impression it makes on the target society.

Fast Facts

Terrorism can not only injure persons physically; the social and psychological impacts on the victims and society can have a longer lasting impact. It can affect them mentally, financially, and their overall connection within a society.

CONCLUSION

Terrorism is not a new concept. The proliferation of terrorism is much easier nowadays with advances in technology and communication. The impact on a society can be prolonged. During and after a terror attack, personal safety must take precedence. The more you protect yourself, the more people you will be able to assist. Everyone in a society can be impacted by the events of terrorism. Proper attention to events, victims, evidence, and care of others can help decrease future attacks.

References

American Nurses Association, & International Association of Forensic Nurses. (2009). *Forensic nursing is the practice of nursing globally when health and legal systems intersect* (p. 3). Silver Spring, MD: Authors.

American Nurses Association, & International Association of Forensic Nursing. (2015). *Forensic nursing scope and standards of practice 2015.* Silver Spring, MD: American Nurses Association.

Blank-Reid, C., & Bokholdt, M. L. (2014). Special populations: The intrapersonal violence trauma patient. In Emergency Nurses Association (Ed.), *TNCC trauma nursing core course provider manual* (7th ed., pp. 283–294). Des Plains, IL: Emergency Nurses Association.

Centers for Disease Control and Prevention. (2018). *Radiological Emergencies (pamphlet).* Atlanta, GA: Author.

Crenshaw, M. (2010). *Terrorism in context* (4th ed.). University Park, PA: Penn State Press.

Eisert, P. J., Elderedge, K., Hartlaub, T., Huggins, E., Keirn, G., O'Brien, P., . . . March, K. S. (2010). CSI: New @ YorkDevelopment of forensic evidence guidelines for the emergency department. *Critical Care Nursing Quarterly, 33*(2), 190–199. doi:10.1097/CNQ.0b013e3181d913b4

Gates, J. D., Arabian, S., Biddinger, P., Blansfield, J., Burke, P., Chung, S., Fischer, J., . . . Yaffe, M. B. (2014). The initial response to the Boston marathon bombing. *Annals of Surgery, 260*(6), 960–966. doi:10.1097/SLA 0000000000000914

Goodwin, R., Kaniasty, K., Sun, S., & Ben-Ezra, M. (2017). Psychological distress and prejudice following terror attacks in France. *Journal of Psychiatric Research, 91*, 111–115. doi:10/1016/j.jpsychires.2017.03.001

Grubbs, T. C. (2014). Preserving crime scene evidence when treating patients at an MCI. *Journal of Emergency Services, 39*, 5.

Holman, E. A., Garfin, D. R., & Silver, R. C. (2014). Media's role in broadcasting acute stress following the Boston Marathon bombings. *Proceedings of the National Academy of Sciences of the United States of America, 111*, 93–98. doi:10.1073/pnas.1316265110

Huey, L. (2015). This is not your mother's terrorism: Social media, online radicalization and the practice of political jamming. *Journal of Terrorism Research, 6*(2). doi:10.15664/jtr.1159

International Military Staff. (2016). NATO's military concept for defence against terrorism. Retrieved from https://www.nato.int/cps/en/natohq/topics_69482.htm

National Institute of Justice. (2000). *A guide for explosion and bombing scene investigation.* Washington, DC: National Institute of Justice.

Okumura, T., Suzuki, K., Fukuda, A., Kohama, A., Takasu, N., Ishimatsu, S., & Hinohara, S. (1998). The Tokyo sarin attack: Disaster management, Part 2: Hospital response. *Academic Emergency Medicine, 5*(6), 618–624. doi:10.1111/j.1553-2712.1998.tb02470.x

Project Management Team. (2014). *After action report for the response to the 2013 Boston Marathon bombings.* Boston: Massachusetts Emergency Management Association.

Thompson, J., Rehn, M., Lossius, H., & Lockey, D. (2014). Risks to emergency responders at terrorist incidents: A narrative review of medical literature. *Critical Care, 18*, 521. doi:10.1186/s13054-014-0521-1

18

Mass Disasters

Corrine Foster and George E. Flores

Sexual violence during and following a disaster is a serious public health issue. Not only does it have catastrophic effects for victims, but it can also be devastating for their community. Nurses who respond to victims of disasters require the necessary knowledge in the complexities of sexual violence during and after disasters so that they can identify and treat patients appropriately.

Upon conclusion of this chapter, the nurse will be able to:

1. State three reasons why the incidences of sexual violence increase during and after disasters.
2. Create a flyer for shelters in a disaster area that promotes awareness of sexual violence, has recommendations for prevention, and lists resources and instructions if an assault is suspected or has occurred.
3. List three recommendations for setting up shelters in a disaster area to improve the safety of vulnerable populations and to mitigate the hazards of sexual violence.

BACKGROUND

Sexual violence can profoundly affect the physical, emotional, mental, and social well-being of victims. It is associated with a number of health consequences, including unwanted pregnancy; gyneco-logical complications such as bleeding, fibroids, chronic pelvic pain, and urinary tract infections; STDs including HIV/AIDS; depression; posttraumatic stress disorder (PTSD); suicidal thoughts and behavior; and reduced quality of life. Research indicates that sexual violence has significant long-term consequences for women's participation in society. One study in Dublin, Ireland, explained the experiences of sexual assault victims, "Fear of crime in general and fear of sexual violence in particular can affect the very nature and quality of women's lives," and that victims of sexual assaults were "more fearful of crime, but they also reported restricting their activities to a greater degree than did male respondents" (Bacik, Maunsell, & Gogan, 1998, pp. 28–30). Healthcare costs of addressing their medical needs are high; in Western Europe alone, sexual assault and DV (domestic violence) "have been estimated to account for 16% of the total health burden" (Bacik, Maunsell, & Gogan, 1998, pp. 28–30). Lost earnings and costs related to victim assistance and the potential loss of ability to care for their families are also critical factors.

Significant and often understudied populations at risk for sexual violence are those displaced by natural disasters. There is a growing body of literature demonstrating the links of sexual violence and those impacted by natural disasters. Below are noted examples:

- Rape of women and children collecting water and firewood has been reported in refugee camps in Guinea and the United Republic of Tanzania (WHO, 2005).Women in refugee camps often are forced to exchange sex for survival needs. As a result, they do not feel safe to go out and gather fuel, food, or clean water for themselves and their families.
- After the 1989 Loma Prieta earthquake in Santa Cruz County, California, reports of sexual violence rose by 300% (Commission for the Prevention of Violence Against Women, 1989).
- Community leaders reported a 31% increase in cases of child sexual abuse and a 21% increase in reported rapes following the Exxon Valdez oil spill in Prince William Sound, Alaska, on March 24, 1989 (Federal Emergency Management Agency [FEMA], 2006).
- A report investigating the social variables surrounding disaster vulnerability (Gender and Post-Disaster Reconstruction: The Case of Hurricane Mitch in Honduras and Nicaragua, 1998) states that a number of shelters witnessed increased sexual violence, coerced prostitution (particularly among adolescent girls), and victimization, leading to physical and psychological trauma (Delaney & Shrader, 2000).

- Both DV and sexual assault were widely reported to increase in the aftermath of the 2004 Indian Ocean tsunami (FEMA, 2006).
- **Hurricane Katrina**: First-hand accounts of the crowded situation in the makeshift shelters in New Orleans tell of the chaos and terror that prevailed there. Many months after Hurricane Katrina, a Texas-based law enforcement official reported, "Many of my investigators and supervisors worked security (in the Superdome and the Convention Center) and were told horror stories by evacuees about what occurred after dark . . . when the people were left without any form of security and roving bands of individuals sexually assaulted victims at will" (Klein, 2008, p. 30).
- Charmaine Neville, famed New Orleans jazz singer and daughter of one of the highly acclaimed Neville Brothers, spoke to the local TV station WAFB a few days after Hurricane Katrina. She described that when she took shelter on the roof of a school after the levees were breached, she was raped by a stranger. She stated in the TV interview, "They put their hand over my mouth, and a knife to my throat, saying, 'If you don't do what I want, I'm gonna kill you and then I'll do what I want to you anyway and throw your body over the side of the building.'"
- **Hurricane Katrina, New Orleans, 2005:** The self-reported incident of rape described in the following text involves a young minority woman looking for food, water, and medicine for her sick elderly mother and her two children: "I was in a [convenience store] with maybe fifty other people looking for medicine for my mama and for water or cokes or anything to drink and candy bars to take to my kids. There was almost nothing left in the store when I got there and I was kind of worried cause there were a lot of drunken young guys starting to tear the place up. They were working on a bank machine [ATM] but couldn't get in it and [were] getting madder and madder. Two of the older ones grabbed me and pulled me in the back of the store and tore my clothes off and raped me one at a time. One held me down in the cooler while the other went at it and then the other took his turn. When they finished the younger one kicked me in the stomach and said 'fuck you, bitch'" The rape victim expressed a sense of fate and resignation with respect to her sexual assault and a belief that reporting the offense to any official agents would serve no purpose (Thornton & Voigt, 2007).
- After Hurricane Katrina 2005, the National Sexual Violence Resource Center (NSVRC) and other organizations developed an anonymous database of self-reported sexual assaults and found that rape crisis centers in cities along the Gulf Coast reported receiving an average of more than 100 calls about incidents of assault and rape from Katrina evacuees. Women and girls accounted for 93% of the victims. Many

more probably occurred but went unreported, since emergency response units and law enforcement agents were stretched thin by countless pressing needs from the public (Firger, 2017).

- A study by Alba and Luciano (2008) identified children as the population most affected by the 2007 Hurricane Noel in the Dominican Republic, determining that they are particularly vulnerable to sexual violence in shelters.

- Kolbe et al. (2010) surveyed 1,800 households in metropolitan Port-au-Prince, Haiti, postearthquake. The authors estimated that over 10,000 people in Port-au-Prince were sexually assaulted during the 6-week period after the earthquake. The authors also found that sexual violence almost exclusively affected women and girls, with almost half of assaults affecting girls under 18 years of age and nearly 3,000 assaults occurring in children under the age of 12 (O'Bryan, 2016).

- The 2012 report "Beyond Shock: Charting the Landscape of Sexual Violence in Post-Quake Haiti," by d'Adesky and PotoFanm+Fi, on sexual violence in the aftermath of the 2010 earthquake in Haiti and the results of a field survey of 2,000 pregnant adolescent girls found that 64% were pregnant as a result of rape, and 37% reported having engaged in transactional or "survival" sex. Additionally, 92% felt that sexual violence/forced sex was more common since the earthquake (O'Bryan, 2016).

- Law enforcement officials are well aware that vulnerable populations are at risk during disasters. Polk County Sheriff Grady Judd posted the following on his official Twitter account (Polk County Sheriff @PolkCoSheriff) just prior to Hurricane Irma: "If you go to a shelter for #Irma, be advised: sworn LEOs will be at every shelter, checking IDs. Sex offenders/predators will not be allowed" (10:30 a.m. —September 6, 2017); "We cannot and we will not have innocent children in a shelter with sexual offenders & predators. Period" (11:16 a.m. —September 6, 2017).

Five reasons sexual violence increases in disasters (Sullivan, 2017):

1. **The Most Vulnerable Are Left Behind**
   Individuals with physical disabilities, the homeless, and those suffering from mental illness or substance abuse are often forced to stay behind while others seek safety from a natural disaster. These individuals are already often targets of sexual violence, but the risk becomes even greater in the aftermath of a disaster.

2. **Crowded Spaces**
   Crowded evacuation shelters expose women and children to an increased risk of sexual assault. Registered sex offenders and families

are sometimes housed in the same building, creating a particularly dangerous situation. Almost a third of reported instances of sexual assault during Hurricane Katrina occurred in evacuation shelters.

3. **Tension and Stress**

During times of disaster, the stress, fear, and sense of helplessness associated with emergency situations tend to increase risk factors for perpetration of violence. As sexual assault is often motivated by a desire for a sense of power and control, a situation that denies everyone of exactly that can lead those who are already prone to violence and abuse to commit additional acts of sexual violence.

4. **An Atmosphere of Chaos**

Police and other emergency personnel are busy addressing the damage caused by the disaster, and those who are around are often not properly trained to deal with reports of sexual assault. People who commit sexual violence then use this chaos to distract from their crimes. Additionally, the emotional turmoil and confusion can make it even more difficult for a victim to respond sufficiently to the situation.

5. **Depleted Resources**

After a disaster, basic resources that can protect people from sexual violence are not readily available. As a result, victims may not be able to seek medical or psychological care or be able to report to law enforcement. For example, shelters that provided a safe haven for those with a sexually abusive partner can be damaged just like any other building. Consequently, the resources and protection they provide can be made temporarily unavailable. Additionally, program staff for rape crisis centers may find themselves displaced as victims of the disaster.

Fast Facts

The most dangerous shelters are those that were understaffed or where staff were not trained in disaster relief.

During and following a disaster, when it is likely that there is an increase in the perpetration of sexual assaults, reporting decreases even more than during times when conditions for reporting are optimal. Completing a medical forensic exam with evidence collection is often difficult with limited resources and personnel. Humanitarian sexual assault evidence collection kits were first developed by Marie Stopes International in 1992, specifically for use during the

Bosnian crisis, when thousands of women were sexually abused and there was an urgent need for appropriate medical equipment. The Sexuality and Family Planning unit of WHO's Regional Office for Europe then reviewed and updated these kits for a second phase in Bosnia. These kits are available through United Nations Population Fund (UNFPA; www.UNFPA.org). However, most medicolegal services are also experiencing chaos during a disaster and are typically unable to respond.

Fast Facts

Regarding Hurricane Katrina evacuation sites: "What you had was a situation where you've got a tremendous amount of vulnerable people, and then some predatory people who had all of the reasons to take their anger out on someone else. Drug and alcohol use is another contributing factor, and no police presence to prevent them from doing whatever they wanted to, to whomever they wanted to" (Judy Benitez, executive director of the Louisiana Foundation Against Sexual Assault; Burnett, 2005).

Fast Facts

Medical triage was being performed at the Houston Astrodome for Hurricane Katrina evacuees, but the process never entailed even a single question about sexual assault. Cassandra Thomas, of the Houston Area Women's Center, was able to add a question about sexual assault to the triage process. However, once the U.S. Department of Homeland Security took over its management, they discontinued all inquiry into sexual victimization or the perpetration of sexual assaults (from an interview with Cassandra Thomas, senior vice president of the Houston Area Women's Center. Houston, TX, on May 15, 2006; Klein, 2008).

Prevention recommendations for shelters and other evacuation sites (from *Sexual Violence in Disasters: A Planning Guide for Prevention and Response*):

- Limit the number of evacuees in each shelter so the population is manageable and can be kept safe.
- Ensure sufficient electrical and/or generator capacity to provide adequate lighting in all public areas.

- Ensure shelters have comprehensive internal and external communication systems including back-up systems. Make sure there is a working public announcement system.
- Provide private spaces for clothing changes and personal hygiene.
- Close off any areas of the shelter space that cannot be made safe and might be conducive to the perpetration of a sexual assault.
- Ensure the presence of adequate, trained law enforcement and other security personnel. Develop a system for involving and screening law enforcement volunteers from other areas.
- Consider the use of closed circuit TV cameras or other surveillance equipment to monitor some areas of the shelter.
- Consider the implementation of "community policing" practices or "floor marshals" so evacuees can look out for each other.
- Consider creating separate sleep and habitation areas for females and males to be used by those who choose to do so. Be especially careful that those with special needs/vulnerable populations are not segregated or that posted information does not increase their vulnerability.
- Consider enforcing a curfew for shelter residents and a "lights out" period during which increased security is available.
- Keep and constantly update comprehensive lists of evacuees, workers, and volunteers in all shelters, including churches, hotels, and arenas:
  - Have all evacuees and workers register as they enter the shelter.
  - Consider issuing picture IDs that must be turned in when evacuees exit the shelter.
  - Issue wristbands to registered shelter residents and staff and allow only individuals with wristbands to enter and exit.
  - Have shelter residents turn in all weapons, for example, knives and guns, upon registration at the shelter.
  - Consider instituting periodic head counts of resident evacuees and shelter staff.
- Implement protocols for how to handle evacuees who are registered sex offenders:
  - Have registered sex offenders report their status as such and consider having them check in with security staff at regular intervals throughout their stay.
  - Have a list of registered sex offenders available for cross-checking evacuees when they register at the shelter.
  - Consider establishing separate emergency shelter sites.

- Provide adequate means of identification for security, law enforcement, and other shelter staff so they can be easily identified by evacuees.
- Ensure that orientations, trainings, and written materials are translated into the appropriate languages.
- In order to ensure that individuals with low literacy skills have access to the sexual violence prevention and response information that can keep them safe, do not rely only on written materials.
- Whenever possible, ensure the availability of hotel suites as emergency shelters for families; this can ease the anxiety of children and allow for greater supervision by parents.
- Ensure provision of basic human needs, for example, adequate food and water, periods of quiet, adequate sleeping arrangements, adequate supplies, and spaces for hygiene and toileting.
- Parents should receive support and instructions concerning their role in the care of and responsibility for their children while in the shelter.
- Create designated areas for children to play that provide safe activities; increase the area's supervision and security. Have trained sexual violence prevention staff screen the individuals who will supervise these areas. Ensure that the physical location does not provide outside access.
- Create designated areas in shelters as safe zones (drug-free zones), play areas, prayer areas, and so on.
- Create designated areas for people in need of mental health services, emergency assistance, and counseling; ensure that they are staffed around the clock by trained mental health professionals.
- Provide an initial mandatory orientation session and regular updates to educate shelter populations, both adults and children, about:
  - Sexual assault and the safety measures they can take to keep themselves and others safe
  - Awareness of one's surroundings, especially the other people in one's immediate vicinity
  - Creating a family safety plan and security for loved ones, especially children and people with disabilities or mental health issues
  - The warning signs or threat of possible perpetration of sexually assaultive or abusive behaviors and how to intervene if necessary
  - Some basic self-defense responses and tactics
  - How to identify shelter security officials and locations as well as safe places that have a constant security presence in place
- Create regular check-ins and meetings for representatives from the various agencies and organizations working within the shelters;

keep lines of communication open between them through the use of walkie-talkies and other devices.

- Ensure regular breaks for shelter staff and volunteers; create opportunities for them to "de-stress."
- Keep evacuees—both adults and children—busy whenever possible with volunteer tasks, entertainment, and other things to occupy their time.
- Develop and distribute a one-page flier and a poster throughout shelters with information about sexual assault, how to prevent it, and what to do in the case of an incident. Try to be location-specific about procedures for reporting and/or seeking assistance.

Fast Facts

Lesbian, gay, bisexual, transgender, queer/questioning, and inter-sex (LGBTQI) are vulnerable populations that are at a heightened risk of trauma, sexual violence, and discrimination during disasters. In one reported case following Katrina, a transperson was jailed after showering in a women's restroom despite being permitted to do so by a volunteer at the relief shelter. "Many of the women who were affected by the storm do not fit the traditional heterosexual image of a 'woman,' and these women not only faced the obstacle of sexism but also homophobia and transphobia as they sought out assistance," writes Charlotte D'Ooge, development director for the American Civil Liberties Union of Louisiana (Thuringer, 2016).

Recommendations when responding to sexual violence (from *Sexual Violence in Disasters: A Planning Guide for Prevention and Response* [Klein, 2008]):

- Ensure that evacuees are supplied with information about how to report an incident of sexual abuse or assault; offer this information in mandatory orientation sessions, updates, and through posters and fliers that are distributed liberally throughout the shelter; ensure materials are in all languages and formats necessary. Encourage evacuees to understand the benefits that seeking services can provide to victims and their loved ones. Assure evacuees that the utmost attention will be given to privacy and confidentiality.
- Ensure that all security, first response staff, volunteers, and other officials in the shelter are briefed on sexual assault response procedures, including whom to contact, where to bring the victim and his or her support people, and how to achieve privacy and confidentiality.

- Train shelter staff and first responders about the possibility that disasters may cause retraumatization for sexual assault survivors and that they may need counseling from rape crisis or other specially trained staff.
- Ensure that private spaces are created for individuals who wish to report sexual assault and seek assistance; have confidential interview rooms available for use by law enforcement and counseling personnel.
- Ensure that each shelter is staffed with a trained sexual assault forensic examiner, that the necessary medical equipment is available for any forensic procedures that may need to be conducted, and that a safe, private space for medical examinations is available at all times.
- Work with the FEMA to establish Disaster Medical Assistance Teams (DMATs) that specialize in sexual violence-related responses, for example, that are able to carry out specialized forensic sexual assault examinations or ensure that every team has at least one member who is certified to conduct forensic exams on a victim of sexual assault.
- Ensure that each shelter is staffed with a trained sexual assault crisis staff person at all times; ensure that this person is contacted immediately if a report of sexual assault is made to anyone working at the emergency site.
- Train law enforcement personnel in how to take reports of sexual violence during disasters, including how to take a "courtesy report" on a sexual assault perpetrated in another district.
- Maintain documentation, including actions taken on behalf of clients; ensure that the documentation is kept in a secure location.
- Create sexual assault support groups for people who may have been victimized or who need help to feel safe; create safe spaces and counseling sessions for previous victims of sexual assault who may feel traumatized by a sense of increased vulnerability because of shelter conditions.

Risk for Human Trafficking

The risk for human trafficking increases in time of natural disasters, as people are displaced and vulnerable. Traffickers exploit the situation, and the activity is rampant in the aftermath of natural disasters. Globally, sites of natural disaster and devastation are recognized as inevitable sites of increased human trafficking, with children being the most vulnerable. After the devastating earthquake in Nepal in 2015, human trafficking shot up by at least 15%, according to a report of the National Human Right Commission of Nepal (NHRC, 2017). Why was this disaster such a perfect opportunity for predators? Traffickers target these vulnerable areas because of the chaos: Children separated from their families (lost, or thought to be dead) can be trafficked among the destruction, without the trafficker being threatened with immediate apprehension. Traffickers prey on desperation and can easily disguise themselves as disaster relief personnel (religious leaders, relief workers, governmental agents, etc.) to arrange transactions with parents (to send their children to better, safer circumstances), only to usher these children into national/transnational rings. Poor, hungry, desperate children, with or without families, can be enticed by financial propositions: the opportunity to work and make money, or send money home to their devastated families (Garsd, 2017).

In an attempt to decrease the incidences of sexual violence on campuses, many colleges are teaching the three Ds of bystander intervention:

- Direct: Directly intervene, in the moment, to prevent a problem situation from happening.
- Delegate: Seek help from another individual, often someone who is authorized to represent others, such as a police officer or campus official.
- Distract: Interrupt the situation without directly confronting the offender.
- Follow the rules for bystander intervention:
  - Do not put yourself at risk.
  - Do not make the situation worse.

CONCLUSION

Disasters have a significant impact on the vulnerability to sexual violence and human trafficking. Those most vulnerable are at a significant risk during the disaster and after the immediacy of the disaster. Nurses who care for victims of disasters should be alerted to the seriousness of sexual violence and help screen and address those who are victims of sexual violence. Future directions of disaster response teams should address the need for forensic nurses who can be instrumental in caring for these victims and providing medical forensic examinations and evidence collection.

References

Alba, W., & Luciano, D. (2008). *Salud sexual y reproductiva y violencia en personas vulnerables: La tormenta Noel en República Dominicana* [Sexual and reproductive health and violence in vulnerable people: Noel Storm in Dominican Republic]. Santo Domingo, Dominican Republic: International Research and Training Institute for the Advancement of Women and United Nations Population Fund.

Bacik, I., Maunsell, C., & Gogan, S. (1998). *The legal process and victims of rape.* Dublin: Cahill Printers Limited.

Burnett, J. (2005, December 21). More stories emerge of rapes in post-Katrina Chaos. *National Public Radio.* Retrieved from https://www.npr.org/templates/story/story.php?storyId=5063796

Commission for the Prevention of Violence Against Women. (1989). *Violence against women in the aftermath of the October 17, 1989 earthquake: A report to the mayor and city council of the city of Santa Cruz.* Santa Cruz, CA: Author.

d'Adesky, A. C. (2012). *Beyond shock: Charting the landscape of sexual violence in post-quake Haiti: Progress, challenges & emerging trends 2010–2012* [en línea].

Delaney, P. L., & Shrader, E. (2000). *Gender and post-disaster reconstruction: The case of Hurricane Mitch in Honduras and Nicaragua. Decision review draft.* Washington, DC: LCSPG/LAC Gender Team, The World Bank.

Federal Emergency Management Agency. (2006). *Violence against women in disasters fact sheet FEMA training handout 20–7: Violence against women in disasters.* Retrieved from http://training.FEMA.gov

Firger, J. (2017, September 10). Hurricanes like Irma increase risk for sexual assault. *Newsweek.* Retrieved from https://www.newsweek.com/hurricane-irma-shelters-sexual-assault-violence-shelters-662558

Garsd, J. (2017, October 5). Human trafficking is a hidden aftermath of natural disasters, Public Radio International's The World. Retrieved from https://www.pri.org/stories/2017-10-05/human-trafficking-hidden-aftermath-natural-disasters

Klein, A. (2008). Sexual violence in disasters: A planning guide for prevention and response, Louisiana Foundation against Sexual Assault & National Sexual Violence Resource Center. Retrieved from https://www.nsvrc.org/publications/nsvrc-publications/sexual-violence-disasters-planning-guide-prevention-and-response

O'Bryan, J., Khoshnood, K., & Lee, B. (2016). *A systematic review of sexual violence and HIV in the post-disaster context: Latin America and the Caribbean.* Retrieved from, ProQuest Dissertations and Theses (1214).

Sullivan, S. (2017). Five reasons sexual violence increases in disasters. *National Violence Resource Center.* Retrieved from https://www.nsvrc.org/blogs/five-reasons-sexual-violence-increases-disasters

Thornton, W. E., & Voigt, L. (2007). Disaster rape: Vulnerability of women to sexual assaults during Hurricane Katrina. *Journal of Public Management and Social Policy, 13*(2), 23–49.

Thuringer, C. (2016). Left out and behind: Fully incorporating gender into the climate discourse. *New Security Beat.* Retrieved from https://www.newsecuritybeat.org/2016/08/left-behind-fully-incorporating-gender-climate-discourse

World Health Organization (WHO). (2005). *Violence and disasters.* Retrieved from http://www.who.int/violence_injury_prevention/publications/violence/violence_disasters.pdf

Index

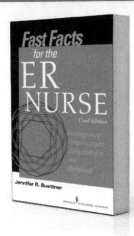
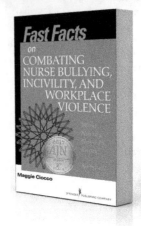
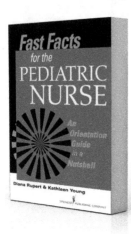
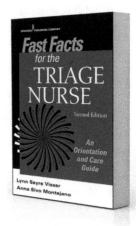

CPSIA information can be obtained
at www.ICGtesting.com
Printed in the USA
BVHW031957260922
648017BV00009B/230